Self-Study Guide
to accompany

Essentials of Nutrition and Diet Therapy

Sixth Edition

Sue Rodwell Williams, Ph.D., M.P.H., R.D.

President, SRW Productions, Inc., and Clinical Nutrition Consultant, Davis, California;
Formerly Metabolic Nutritionist, Kaiser-Permanente Northern California
Regional Newborn Screening and Metabolic Program,
Director, Clinical Nutrition and ADA Traineeship Program in Dietetics,
Kaiser-Permanente Medical Center, Oakland, California;
and Field Faculty, M.P.H.-Dietetic Internship Program
and Coordinated Undergraduate Program in Dietetics,
University of California, Berkeley

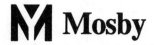 Mosby

St. Louis Baltimore Boston Chicago London Madrid Philadelphia Sydney Toronto

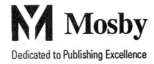

Mosby

Dedicated to Publishing Excellence

94 95 96 97 98   /PC   9 8 7 6 5 4 3 2 1

PREFACE

Throughout its previous editions, this little study guide has aided many students in their beginning and review study of basic clinically-oriented nutrition. This fundamental goal remains paramount in this new sixth edition. It is designed to accompany my new textbook editions and reflect their expanded scope and approach to a broadened nutritional science base and changing health care attitudes and practices, both public and professional. Its chapter divisions are correlated with those in the sixth edition of *Essentials of Nutrition and Diet Therapy*. However, the general study structure may also be useful for many students using the seventh edition of my more advanced text, *Nutrition and Diet Therapy*.

Major Changes in this Edition

As the companion to my introductory clinically-oriented textbook, *Essentials of Nutrition and Diet Therapy*, this study guide follows closely the major changes in the new edition of the text. A number of correlations appear here:

1. Reorganization of Material

Following the revised material of the *Essentials* text, the material in the study guide has been reorganized to combine some chapters and make way for several new ones. These changes are intended to facilitate your learning and lay an initial foundation for sound clinical practice.

2. New Chapters

Several new chapters, and new sections of previous ones, reflect new material added to the corresponding *Essentials* text. Chapters 18 and 24 are completely new, reviewing current practices in: (1) alternative feeding methods of enteral and parenteral nutrition support, and (2) rapid advances in knowledge of AIDS, the evolution of its causative virus, and current medical/nutritional management. Chapter 6 combines two previous chapters -- the background physiology of energy balance and its practical application to newer personal and individual health approaches in weight management. Chapter 13 includes a more balanced approach to adult nutrition with additional material on the young and middle adult years. Chapter 20 provides a more comprehensive integrated overview of the circulatory system and its clinical problems in diseases of the heart, blood vessels, and lungs. Chapter 26 expands its view of disabling diseases to include major sections on musculoskeletal disease, neuromuscular disease, and progressive neurologic disorders. New summary-review material, self-test items, and learning activities review these new chapters and sections.

3. <u>New Book Format and Design</u>

To help students in their learning of new subject matter, this edition matches the new format and design of its accompanying *Essentials* text. Its form is easy to follow and heightens interest and learning.

4. <u>New Learning Aids</u>

As in previous editions, this new revision of the study guide applies a number of the learning aids in the *Essentials* text. The many text references and boxes expand nutrition knowledge and skills in current practice, address current nutrition-related issues and controversies, and provide background for this self-test review of comprehensive learning.

5. <u>New Study Guide Sections</u>

Following the revised format of the *Essentials* text, the chapter sections are reflected in this accompanying study guide. At the beginning of each chapter a Chapter Focus presents the major principles and concepts that the chapter develops. This brief statement targets the chapter's overall goal or purpose. Then throughout the self-test sections directions are given to guide the student's responses and point to use of the Test Key in the Appendix. Finally, each chapter concludes with a section on Current Nutrition Issues that focuses student attention on a related article in the accompanying textbook. There several thought-provoking questions help the student explore the issue developed in the article.

6. <u>New Answer Key Expansion</u>

The study guide Appendix provides a comprehensive answer key, updating chapters and providing new testing material for the new and expanded chapters outlined above. Here, each true-false and multiple-choice test item answer carries a statement of its rationale. Thus this key helps the student not only to know the correct answer but also to understand *why* it is the correct answer. This item analysis will reinforce and strengthen the learning process.

7. <u>Enhanced Readability and Student Interest</u>

As with the accompanying *Essentials* text, much of the study guide has been rewritten to draw students into the material and facilitate learning, with a format and writing style designed to capture interest and a comprehensive content to present basic sound information that can be easily understood. Many issues of student, public, and professional interest are tested and reviewed. All the topics have current relevance to help clarify questions and concerns.

Additional Changes New to this Edition

In addition to these main changes, I have made substantive changes to relate this guide to its new accompanying *Essentials* text:

1. Summary-Review Quizzes

This initial section of each chapter has been updated and organized to reflect new and reorganized material in the *Essentials* text chapters. The introductory paragraph gives the student specific directions for filling in the blanks in each review section from list of numbered responses following. The overall section material is divided into smaller subsections to focus on contributing principles, with an accompanying brief list of fill-in words and phrases to complete each section of review statements. This entire completed review section then provides an outline of the chapter highlights.

2. Discussion Questions

This brief section is updated and revised to stimulate thinking about the text material, especially its application to modern health-related issues.

3. Self-Test Questions

In both the true-false and multiple-choice subsections, there are new and revised items reflecting the updated and new text material. These test items provide experience in analyzing material on similar test items in examinations.

4. Learning Activities

This practical section of each chapter includes the new and updated accompanying text material. Numerous activities are outlined for individual and group projects in the classroom, the home, the community, and clinical areas.

How to Use This Study Guide: A Note to Students

A basic skill in any science is that of problem-solving through the development of logical steps to find reasonable solutions. This process also applies to nutritional science and its use in human health care. This study guide is organized to facilitate your study in these areas in several ways:

- To help you focus your immediate attention on the main concepts in the chapter topic

- To help you summarize and review the main points in each chapter

- To encourage and stimulate your thinking about several key issues and questions related to the chapter material

- To help you test your own understanding of the basic text chapter

- To apply concepts and principles involved, through the use of case problems, individual and group learning activities, experiments, and projects

- To illustrate the chapter topic by a related current nutrition issue and the questions it may raise in your own mind

Thus each chapter consists of six sections: (1) *Chapter Focus*, setting forth key concepts involved; (2) *Summary-Review Quiz*, outlining chapter highlights; (3) *Discussion Questions*, stimulating further thought about key chapter concepts; (4) *Self-Test Questions*, analyzing both true-false and multiple-choice items; (5) *Learning Activities*, leading to exploration and applications of principles learned; and (6) *Current Nutrition Issues*, providing inquiry questions concerning *Issues and Answers* articles in the text. Look at these sections and consider how they may help meet your learning needs.

Remember the learning process sequence:

1. Read the related chapter carefully. See it first as a whole, then in its organized parts, and finally as a whole again, enhanced now by a greater understanding of each part.

2. Review your class notes, and any additional outside research notes.

3. If there is any part you don't understand of your text chapter or your class/research notes, seek help immediately, either from your instructor or your student study group.

4. Test your understanding of each text chapter using the corresponding chapter in your study guide.

Chapter focus First read this concise statement incorporating the major concepts of the chapter topic. Does it bring clearly to your mind the key ideas involved?

Summary-review quiz Complete this first section immediately after you have read the related text chapter carefully. This review activity will help you gain, first, a broad view of the principles and general information presented. Then, as you proceed, each summary-review quiz provides the background for grasping the developing material in subsequent chapters. To complete each quiz, choose the correct word or phrase for each blank from the list provided in each subsection. Write both the word or phrase and its number in the corresponding blank.

Discussion questions These questions provide a more intensive digging into a few selected topics or issues related to the text discussion. They will help you organize your thinking about problems raised in each chapter and give you valuable practice in writing essay examinations. Think about each question carefully and reread pertinent portions of the text as needed. Then write out your answer clearly and completely in logical sequence of ideas. You may use these questions to explore ideas individually or as a basis for discussion in small groups.

At this point, to explore these questions more deeply, you may want to consult additional references. Look over the references suggested in your textbook. It is always a good habit to consult references in addition to your text for a broader range of comparative data and their applications. Remember that a lifetime of learning comes only from forming early the habit of asking questions about everything you hear, read, or observe -- especially questions of "how?", "why?", and "so what?" In other words, *think* about what you read and ask questions constantly.

Self-test questions Here you can narrow your study to specific facts and conclusions. Test your knowledge of the basic content presented. Respond to each self-test item in two ways. First, go through each of the true-false statements, circle either the T or F before each item, and then write a brief statement giving the reason for the correct answer. Second, go through each of the multiple-choice items in the same manner, circling the letter before the answer you choose and writing a brief reason for your answer. Now, after having completed both parts, turn to the answer key in the Appendix and check your answers. Note the brief reasons for the correct answer in the key and be sure you understand each item, especially those that you have answered incorrectly or those of which you are unsure.

Current nutrition issues In this final section you will find inquiry questions to guide your thinking about an *Issues and Answers* article in your accompanying *Essentials* text. First, read the indicated article carefully. As you read, consider the questions it raises in your own mind or any feelings you may have about the issue. Then answer each of the questions according to your own personal response to the article. In your written response try to organize and express your ideas logically. This will provide further practice in developing answers to essay questions on examinations.

A Note To Instructors

The last two sections described above may provide suggestions for planning course work or class projects and assignments. In the section on learning activities you may find some types of activities appropriate for your teaching situation or needs, or related to skills that need developing. Active participation in problem-solving activities leads to effective learning. Some of these activities are individual and some are group projects. Some may be done in the classroom, whereas many may be carried out at home or in the community or clinical area. In each instance, the key principles involved will acquire more meaning through active student participation. Also, you may find that a particular *Issues and Answers* article that is the focus of the Current Nutrition Issues section may be pertinent to your teaching goals and provide a basis for stimulating class discussion on this particular issue.

Acknowledgements

Many persons have helped me in developing this new study guide edition to make it more useful in student learning. To these persons I give my thanks: to my publisher, editorial staff, and book production crew at Mosby for their skill and constant support; to those teachers who gave valuable reviewer suggestions; to my own staff for their usual skillful research, manuscript production, and personal help with innumerable tasks; to my many students, interns, colleagues, clients, and patients who have always been my constant teachers; and to my family who always shares in whatever I am able to achieve.

Sue Rodwell Williams
Davis, California

CONTENTS

Chapter 1
NUTRITION AND HEALTH

Chapter Focus

Human nutrition and health around our world are inevitably linked. They relate to the physical, political, and human environments as well as to the rapid advance of science and technology, both of which are rapidly changing our society. Thus health maintenance and disease control demand team care at all levels, based on human concern for human needs.

Summary-Review Quiz

Fill in the blanks below with the appropriate number and word(s) from the list following each section. Each numbered word is used; some may be used more than once. When you've completed all the sections, check your answers for each blank against the test key. Correct any mistakes and then review the entire chapter summary.

1. The science of nutrition is based on the physical sciences of _____, which describes the chemical nature of nutrients and their fate in the body, and _____, which shows how these nutrients work together to achieve _____ of the whole body. This highly sensitive level of internal control is called _____. In addition, the _____ sciences show psychosocial and economic influences that help us understand who we are and how our food habits relate to human development.

2. The macronutrients _____ and _____ supply the main sources of energy and _____ mainly supplies the structural units _____ for building tissue. Smaller amounts of the micronutrients _____ and _____ regulate body processes. The additional nutrients _____ and _____ also act as significant regulatory agents. The term _____ covers the sum of all the body's chemical processes that sustain life.

1. orderly functioning
2. vitamins
3. metabolism
4. behavioral sciences
5. dietary fiber
6. physiology
7. protein
8. homeostasis
9. minerals
10. fats
11. water
12. biochemistry
13. carbohydrates
14. amino acids

3. In our rapidly changing world, current major U.S. health problems focus on chronic disease: _____ disease, _____ in various forms, and complications of _____ and _____ disease. At all levels of health care—world, national, state, and local community—only a _____ approach that is both preventive and person-centered can be effective.

4.   In modern health care, we confront new and different problems based on new lifestyles, _____, _____, changing values and community patterns, _____, and environmental _____. Therefore the fundamental framework for the study of basic nutrition must be built on the learning concepts of _____ and _____.

1. social issues
2. cancer
3. renal
4. balance
5. team

6. malnutrition
7. diabetes mellitus
8. change
9. heart
10. economic stress

11. pollution

5.   Formerly, and to some extent even now, the basic approach to care has been _____, with training of hospital and community workers centered on skills for treating _____.   Currently, however, education in the health fields is based on a _____ approach and on a _____ concept of _____ or wellness, rather than a _____ concept of _____, or illness. This new approach values _____ beyond mere physical survival.

6. Two main factors have brought about these changes in health values and practices. These factors are the rapid increase in _____ and in _____, both of which have caused rapid social change. Problems have resulted, however. Increased "know-how" has brought more specialization and higher _____. An increased number of people and an increased length of life have brought a greater increase in the _____ of aging.

1. positive
2. negative
3. scientific knowledge
4. chronic illnesses
5. health

6. curative
7. disease
8. population
9. preventive
10. medical care costs

11. quality of life

7. Changes must occur, therefore, in ways of providing health care. These include: (1) changes that focus on the _____ involved as root causes of disease, malnutrition, and illness; (2) changes in health care systems to include more _____ in a variety of hospital and _____ and community health centers; (3) changes in the role of the _____, or health client, to include active involvement in personal health needs through better nutrition and health education; and (4) changes in methods of _____ to include some form of health insurance to meet mounting costs.

8. The rapidly changing _____ and increased _____ and action have contributed to new priorities and needs in nutritional therapy and education. Attention has been focused on problems of _____, especially in poverty areas, and on the _____ persons in our population.

9. In the light of these problems, then, nutrition must be defined in terms of what it does toward _____ . Nutrition is specifically related to both _____ and _____ health and well-being.

1. patient	6. malnutrition	11. social issues
2. consumer awareness	7. aging	12. payment for services
3. physical	8. special clinic settings	
4. meeting human need	9. food environment	
5. health team care	10. psychosocial	

Discussion Questions

1. Why are mutual interaction and dependency among the countries of the world becoming increasingly important in solving world nutrition and health problems?

2. What is your own present definition of nutrition?

3. How do you think nutrition relates to the health of individuals and groups? What personal observations can you give to support your statement?

4. Explain the meaning of the statement: "Food habits do not develop in a vacuum."

5. Describe and compare the three types of U.S. nutritional guides: (1) nutrient standards, (2) food guides, and (3) health promotion guidelines. How may these tools be used to support sound nutrition? Can they also be misused? How? Illustrate you answer.

Self-Test Questions

True-False
Circle the "T" if a statement is true and write a brief rationale for its accuracy. If it is false, circle the "F" and write the correct statement.

T F 1. American society tends to be youth- and action-oriented and therefore often isolates and devalues its elderly citizens.

T F 2. Food habits are closely related to cultural influences and psychosocial development.

T F 3. The American population has increased greatly in the past few decades, but its general characteristics remain essentially the same today.

T F 4. Nutrients work independently in the body.

T F 5. Food processing has little influence on the amount of nutrients in the food or on its safety, appearance, and taste.

T F 6. Certain foods are called *complete foods* because they contain all the nutrients needed for full growth and health.

Multiple Choice

Circle the letter in front of the correct answer. Then check your answers by the test key (p 243). Now compare all the possible answers for each item and write the following brief statements: (1) rationale for the correct answer, and (2) why each of the other responses is incorrect.

1. All persons throughout life have need for:
   a. the same amount of nutrients at any age
   b. the same nutrients but in varying amounts
   c. the same amount of nutrients in any state of health
   d. different nutrients in varying amounts

2. Nutrients are:
   a. foods necessary for good health
   b. chemical compounds or elements in foods having specific metabolic functions
   c. nourishments used to cure certain illnesses
   d. metabolic control agents such as enzymes

3. Specific nutrients needed by the body:
   a. are available through food in a variety of combinations
   b. must usually be obtained by additional pills or supplements
   c. must be obtained by specific food combinations
   d. do not have specific functions but can be used in a variety of ways

Learning Activities
Community Nutrition Assessment

1. What problems do you see in your environment that are related to nutrition? Consider environment as broadly as you wish—local community, general area, state, country, or world.

2.   Pick one of the problems you noted above. What kinds of information do you need to find some solutions to this problem? Where would you search? What resources—places, persons, or reference materials—would you use?

3.   At this point what solutions to this problem can you see? Give any reasons or evidence that you can think of to support your solutions.

Personal Nutrition Assessment
   Select a specific person as a subject. Observe this person carefully and make a general assessment of individual signs of nutritional status. For a reference guide, use Table 1-1: Clinical Signs of Nutritional Status, *Essentials of Nutrition and Diet Therapy*, ed 6, p 7; *Nutrition and Diet Therapy*, ed 7, p 7).

Current Nutrition Issues
   Read carefully the *Issues and Answers* article, "If You're Not Healthy, It's Your Own Fault!" (*Essentials of Nutrition and Diet Therapy*, ed 6, p 16; *Nutrition and Diet Therapy*, ed 7, p 17). Consider these inquiry questions:

1. Why would such an attitude of individual blame for personal health problems arise at all in some persons' minds?

2. What do you think is right or wrong with this accusation? Give some examples to support your view.

3. How may concerned health workers overcome this attitude of blame? What positive health care actions can they follow with their clients?

4. In turn, what do you think would be the most helpful health care role for clients or patients to follow?

Chapter 2
CARBOHYDRATES

Chapter Focus

The nature of carbohydrate—its wide availability, storage capacity, and relatively low cost as a food—make it our major fuel source. Our bodies rapidly cycle starches and sugars to provide needed energy.

Summary-Review Quiz

Fill in the blanks below with the appropriate number and word(s) from the list following each section. Each numbered word is used; some may be used more than once. When you've completed all the sections, check your answers for each blank against the test key. Correct any mistakes and then review the entire chapter summary.

1. The primary survival task of the human body is that of securing _____ to do its work. As "raw" fuel, _____ must be changed to the usable refined fuel _____, which is then carried to the site of _____ in the cells, where it can be burned.

2. In the human energy system the major dietary source of quick energy is _____. This stored fuel is found in plant foods as _____ and _____. Plants transform energy from the sun, using _____ and _____ as raw materials, and _____ in green leaves as a catalyst to manufacture this potential energy. The name *carbohydrate* comes from its structural chemical elements _____, _____, and _____.

1. carbon	6. oxygen	11. energy production
2. carbohydrate	7. starches	12. chlorophyll
3. carbon dioxide	8. water	13. glucose
4. sugars	9. energy	
5. carbohydrate foods	10. hydrogen	

3. The simplest form of carbohydrate is a _____. Three of these simple sugars important in human nutrition are _____, _____, and _____. The somewhat more complex double sugars are called _____. The three main double sugars are _____, _____, and _____. Still more complex dietary carbohydrates made up of many sugar units are the _____. Two of these complex carbohydrates are important in human nutrition: _____ as a major energy source and _____ as needed bulk and binding agents.

4. A relatively small amount of body carbohydrate is stored in the _____ and muscles in the form of _____. The _____ constantly carries a small additional amount. Therefore, _____ is needed regularly to meet energy demands and to spare _____ from being used too much for energy. Also sufficient carbohydrate has an _____, thus preventing too rapid a breakdown of fat for energy, with the resulting accumulation in the blood of strong acids called

_____.

1. disaccharides	7. dietary carbohydrate	13. monosaccharide
2. polysaccharides	8. lactose	14. starches
3. dietary fiber	9. protein	15. galactose
4. antiketogenic effect	10. ketones	16. glycogen
5. liver	11. blood sugar	17. fructose
6. glucose	12. sucrose	18. maltose

5. Two vital body organs are especially dependent on a constant supply of carbohydrate in the form of _____ to supply energy to operate their specific functions. These organs are the _____ and the _____.

6. The refined fuel used by the cells for making energy available for body work is _____. It is produced from food carbohydrate by the combined action of _____ and _____ digestion. As a result of this combined action, the _____ are produced and absorbed in the _____, then carried directly in the portal blood system to the tissues.

7. The _____ are the energy production sites. Here the refined fuel _____ is broken down to release stored _____ for cell work through a series of _____ chemical reactions. This overall system of chemical processes by which energy is made available for the body is called _____. A special chemical compound produced anywhere along the way by these many special metabolic processes is called a _____.

1. mechanical	6. brain	11. enzyme-controlled
2. cells	7. potential energy	12. glucose
3. heart	8. metabolite	
4. small intestine	9. simple sugars	
5. metabolism	10. chemical	

Discussion Questions

1. What kind of sugar is in the blood? How does it differ from the sugar in the sugar bowl?

2. Where does blood sugar come from? Only from sugar?

3. What is the "sugar phobia syndrome" observed among some persons? Why do you think it has developed? Are these fears justified? Give examples to support your answer.

4. From your general observation and experience do you see any trends in form and amount of carbohydrate used in the American diet?

Self-Test Questions

True-False
Circle the "T" if a statement is true and write a brief rationale for its accuracy. If it is false, circle the "F" and write the correct statement.

T F 1. Carbohydrates are composed of carbon, hydrogen, oxygen, and nitrogen.
T F 2. The main carbohydrate food in our diet is starch.
T F 3. Modern processing and refinement of our foods has reduced the amount of fiber in our diet.
T F 4. Lactose is a very sweet simple sugar found free in a number of carbohydrate foods.
T F 5. Glucose is the form in which sugar circulates in the blood.
T F 6. A small amount of the fiber in foods that we eat is digested, but the major portion is carried through the body and provides important bulk in the gastrointestinal tract.
T F 7. Glycogen is an important long-term storage form of energy because relatively large amounts of it are deposited in the liver and muscles.

Multiple Choice
Circle the letter in front of the correct answer. Then check your answers by the test key (p 244). Now compare all the possible answers for each item and write the following brief statements: (1) rationale for the correct answer and (2) why each one of the other responses is incorrect.

1. Carbohydrates provide one of the main fuel sources for energy. Which of the following carbohydrate foods provides the *quickest* source of energy?
   a. slice of bread
   b. orange juice
   c. chocolate candy bar
   d. milk

2. The most nutritionally significant refined fuel form of carbohydrate is:
   a. maltose
   b. dextrins
   c. starch
   d. glucose

3. Most of the work of changing food carbohydrate to the refined fuel form glucose is accomplished by enzymes located in the:
   a. mouth
   b. stomach
   c. small intestine
   d. large intestine

4. An adult intolerance to milk, found mostly in Black and Oriental populations, is caused by genetic deficiency of the enzyme:
   a. sucrase
   b. lactase
   c. maltase
   d. amylase

5. Chemical digestion of carbohydrates is completed in the small intestine by enzymes from the:
   a. pancreas and gallbladder
   b. gallbladder and liver
   c. small intestine and pancreas
   d. liver and small intestine

6. A quickly available form of energy, although limited in amount, is stored in the liver by conversion of glucose to:
   a. glycogen
   b. glycerol
   c. tissue fat
   d. amino acids

Learning Activities

Individual or Group Experiment: Initial Carbohydrate Enzyme Digestion
Materials A large sour pickle, some saltine crackers, a cookie, a saucer, a glass of drinking water, and a timer or watch with a second hand.
Procedure Carry out this activity apart from meals or the eating of other food or snacks:

1. Place sour pickle on a saucer, focus your entire attention on it for a brief period and think about its taste and texture. Do you feel anything happening in your mouth or under your jaws?
2. Take a bite of the pickle an hold it in your mouth: then chew slowly and swallow. Does the taste change or remain the same?
3. Drink some water to clear your mouth.
4. Take a large bite of saltine cracker, chew it normally and swallow. Does any taste change occur during this process?
5. Take a second large bite of cracker, then chew it *slowly* for a full minute. Is there any taste change during this time? What is the texture and feel of the food mass in your mouth?
6. Take a bite of the cookie and chew it normally, then swallow. How does it taste?

Results   In each case, describe your responses to the actions and questions given previously.

Discussion
1. What mechanical digestion takes place in the mouth? What is its purpose?

2. What digestive secretions are present in the mouth? Where do they come from? What is their function?

3. Why does so little chemical digestion actually occur in the mouth?

4. Account for the difference in taste of the cracker and the cookie. What are the respective forms of carbohydrate in each?

Situational Problem: Energy
Dick Smith, 21-year-old student, has diabetes. He gives himself an injection of insulin every morning. He is usually active in college athletics, but this is final examination week and he is putting in long hours of study. On the day before a particularly difficult examination, he is anxiously reviewing his study materials at home and forgets to eat lunch. About midafternoon he begins to feel faint and realizes that his blood sugar is low and an insulin reaction is approaching if he does not get a quick source of energy. He looks in the kitchen and all that he can find is orange juice, milk, butter, a loaf of bread, and a jar of peanut butter.

1. Which of these foods should he eat *first*, immediately?

2. Why did you make the choice you did above?

Later, when Dick is feeling better, he makes a peanut butter and butter sandwich, pours a glass of milk, and eats his snack while he continues studying.

3. What carbohydrate sources of energy are in his snack?

4. Are these sources in a form the cell can burn for energy? What changes must his body make in these sources then to get them into the necessary form? What is this usable form of blood sugar?

5. What important relationship do carbohydrate and fat have in the final production of energy in the body? If Dick does not take his insulin to provide the necessary control agent for metabolizing the carbohydrate, what would happen to him as a result of improper handling of fat and the resulting accumulation of ketones?

Individual Diet Analysis

Record in detail your food intake for a day, including meals and snack items. Use the Daily Food Intake box on p 291 to list your day's food, checking each of the carbohydrate items and tracing what happens to them in your body.

Current Nutrition Issues

Read carefully the Clinical Application box, "Hypoglycemia: Fact or Fancy?" (*Essentials of Nutrition and Diet Therapy*, ed 6, p 36; *Nutrition and Diet Therapy*, ed 7, p 46). Consider these inquiry questions:

1. Why do you think such a controversy exists about hypoglycemia?

2.   After comparing the nature and causes of the two types of hypoglycemia, why do you think public opinion has attributed "low blood sugar" to what may be considered excessive amounts of sugar in the diet, with labels such as "sugar blues" or states of "sugar phobia?"

3.   Do you think stress may contribute to this condition? If so, how?

4.   How do the public and professional views regarding diagnosis and treatment differ? What problems are there with extreme views on both sides? How do you think these problems may be avoided?

Chapter 3
FATS

Chapter Focus

Lipids are vital substances in human nutrition, supplying energy and various membrane and metabolic components. But problems related to vascular disease may be associated with excessive amounts.

Summary-Review Quiz

Fill in the blanks below with the appropriate number and word(s) from the list following each section. Each numbered word is used; some may be used more than once. When you've completed all the sections, check your answers for each blank against the test key. Correct any mistakes and then review the entire chapter summary.

1. The fats are important fuels because they are a _____ source of energy and have an almost unlimited body storage capacity in the form of _____ tissue. Fats belong to a class of fats and fat-related compounds called _____.

2. Food fats include such obvious _____ forms as those in bacon, cream, margarine, or oil and more hidden forms such as those in _____ and egg yolk, as well as in plant sources such as _____, avocados, and olives.

3. Fat is composed of the same elements as those in carbohydrates--_____, _____, and _____. However, because fat is much more concentrated a fuel, it provides better than _____ the amount of energy as the same amount of carbohydrate would provide. However, it is not as _____ a source of energy as is carbohydrate but is more a _____ form of energy.

1. carbon	6. concentrated	11. twice
2. quick	7. lipids	12. oxygen
3. visible	8. lean meat	
4. storage	9. hydrogen	
5. nuts	10. adipose fat	

4. The basic structural units of fats are the _____. As with carbohydrate, these units are also made up of the basic chemical elements _____, _____, and _____. They are the key refined fuel form of fat that cells burn for _____.

5. These fat units may be _____ or _____, depending on the number of hydrogen atoms that they contain. The _____, which contain all the hydrogen they can take (filling every available carbon bond), are said to be completely _____. Food fats composed mainly of such units are called _____ and come mainly from _____. Those units with fewer hydrogen atoms are _____. If a fat unit has only one such unfilled spot, it is called a _____. If it has two or more unfilled places in its structure, it is called a _____. Food fats composed mainly of such unfilled units are called _____ and come from _____.

1. saturated fats	6. monounsaturated fatty acid	11. animal sources
2. unsaturated fatty acids	7. carbon	12. fatty acids
3. saturated	8. plant sources	13. oxygen
4. polyunsaturated fatty acids	9. unsaturated fats	14. energy
5. hydrogen	10. unsaturated	15. saturated fatty acids

6. The main essential fatty acid is _____. It helps to lower _____, build tissue _____, prolong _____ time, and form _____, groups of local hormone-like compounds active in body tissues. The most widespread of these compounds in tissue actions are called _____. The main essential fatty acid must be included in the _____, since the body cannot produce it. Its main food sources are _____.

7. Whether in food or in the body, basic dietary and tissue fats are _____. This name indicates the chemical structure: a _____ base with three _____ attached.

1. glycerol	6. triglycerides	11. prostaglandins
2. blood-clotting	7. linoleic acid	
3. diet	8. vegetable oils	
4. serum cholesterol	9. membranes	
5. fatty acids	10. eicosanoids	

8. Food fats are changed to the refined fuel form, the _____, through the process of _____ that takes place mainly in the _____ by the enzyme action of _____ with the aid of the emulsifying agent _____. The process is incomplete in the intestine itself but is completed within the cells of the intestinal wall by the enzyme _____.

9. The initial products of fat digestion, although incomplete, are absorbed from the intestine into the _____ of the intestinal wall by combination with _____ as a carrier. Here, after the digestive breakdown is completed, new _____ are reformed from the _____ and an active form of _____ for use by the body as fat. These newly formed _____ are combined with a small amount of _____ as the carrier to form _____ called _____.

10. These initial post-meal transport forms of fat, the _____, are then absorbed first into the _____ system and travel via the portal blood system to the _____. Here, after conversion to other carrier _____ of less heavy fat loads, the fat is carried to all body tissue for use as _____ or to _____ tissue for storage and release as needed.

1. enteric lipase
2. triglycerides
3. adipose fat
4. lipoproteins
5. mucosal cells
6. pancreatic lipase

7. lymphatic
8. protein
9. liver
10. fatty acids
11. energy
12. chylomicrons

13. small intestine
14. glycerol
15. digestion
16. bile

11. In human nutrition, the _____ are important classes of fat carriers. Fat cannot travel free in the blood because it is _____ in water; so this combination is the main _____ form of fat in the blood stream. In the underlying disease process in heart disease—_____—some forms of these blood lipids may be elevated and thus add a _____ for the development of _____.

12. Though not a fat itself, another important complex fat-related compound found in almost all body tissue is _____. Because of its vital metabolic functions it is synthesized in the body, mainly in the _____. It is also consumed in foods, such as _____ and organ meats, both of which contain large amounts. Elevated levels of _____ have also been associated with _____ and its underlying pathology _____.

13. The vital fat-related compound _____ also has an important metabolic function as precursor of _____, which is made from a form of the compound in the _____ on exposure to _____. It is also closely associated with other steroid compounds such as sex and adrenal _____.

1. atherosclerosis
2. sunlight
3. cardiovascular disease
4. cholesterol
5. insoluble

6. egg yolk
7. serum cholesterol
8. skin
9. liver
10. lipoproteins

11. risk factor
12. transport
13. vitamin D
14. hormones

Discussion Questions

1. Describe the fat component of the present American diet in terms of amount and kind. What general modifications are desirable for health? Why?

2.   Why can fat never travel free in the blood? Why does protein serve as a good carrier? What are these resulting carrier compounds?

3.   Define cholesterol and saturated fats. How are they associated with atherosclerosis?

4.   Define omega-3 fatty acids and eicosanoids. Why is so much current research being focused on these compounds?

5.   How is margarine made into a food fat similar to butter in texture and nutrition? How does margarine differ from butter? Are there any concerns about our increased consumption of margarine in place of butter?

6.   What relation does chain length of fatty acids have to their absorption? What is the commercial product MCT? What is it used for?

Self-Test Questions

<u>True-False</u>
        Circle the "T" if a statement is true and write a brief rationale for its accuracy. If it is false, circle the "F" and write the correct statement.

T F 1.   Although the body synthesizes cholesterol daily, dietary cholesterol also affects serum cholesterol and hence is restricted in treatment for elevated blood lipids.

T F 2.   Corn oil is a saturated fat.

T F 3.   Polyunsaturated fats usually come from animal sources.

T F 4.   Increased amounts of foods containing linoleic acid are desirable in the diet of the person having elevated serum cholesterol.

T F 5.   Bile helps to digest fats through its powerful enzyme action.

T F 6.   The final end products of fat digestion are glycogen and fatty acids.

T F 7.   Lipoproteins are transport forms of triglycerides and cholesterol produced mainly in the intestinal wall and in the liver.

T F   8.   Fat has approximately the same caloric value as carbohydrate.

Multiple Choice
 Circle the letter in front of the correct answer. Then check your answers by the test key (p 245). Now compare all the possible answers for each item and write the following brief statements: (1) rationale for the correct answer and (2) why each one of the other responses is incorrect.

1. The fuel form of fat found in food sources is:
 a. triglyceride
 b. fatty acid
 c. glycerol
 d. lipoprotein

2. Which of the following statements are correct concerning the saturation of fats?
 (1) The degree of saturation depends on the relative amount of hydrogen in the component fatty acid.
 (2) The more unsaturated fats come from animal sources.
 (3) The more saturated the fat, the softer it tends to be.
 (4) Fats composed of fatty acids with two or more double bonds in their carbon chains are called *polyunsaturated*.
 a. 1 and 2
 b. 3 and 4
 c. 1 and 4
 d. 2 and 4

3. A therapeutic diet frequently used in the treatment of heart disease is the low-saturated fat diet. Which of the following foods would be allowed on this diet?
 a. whole milk
 b. oil-vinegar salad dressing
 c. butter
 d. cheddar cheese

4. An important material produced in the liver and stored in the gallbladder is needed to prepare food fats for change to usable fuel forms. This material is:
 a. lipase
 b. amylase
 c. bile
 d. cholesterol

5. The major digestive changes in fat are accomplished in the small intestine by a lipase from the pancreas. This enzymatic activity:
 a. because of its strength, easily breaks down all the dietary fat to fatty acids and glycerol
 b. because of the difficulty of this reaction, splits off all the fatty acids in only about 25% of the total dietary fat consumed
 c. synthesizes new triglycerides from the dietary fat consumed
 d. emulsifies the fat globules and reduces their surface tension

18

Learning Activities

Individual or Group Experiment: Fat Solubility in Water

Materials Water, liquid vegetable oil, prepared mustard (not dry mustard power), small glass jars with lids, small bowl, and liquid detergent.

Procedure

1. In one of the jars place equal parts of water and oil. Secure the lid and shake vigorously.
2. Place the jar on a flat surface and let it remain still. Observe the mixture carefully.
3. Repeat the above procedure in the second jar, but this time add 1 tablespoon of prepared mustard. Secure the lid and shake vigorously.
4. Place the second jar beside the first one and let it remain still. Observe the mixture carefully.
5. In a small bowl, pour some water and add one tablespoon of oil. Add one tablespoon of liquid detergent, dropping it a small amount at a time on the surface of the water and oil mixture. Observe any changes that occur.

Results

1. What happens to the water-fat mixture on standing? Why?

2. What happens to the water-fat-mustard mixture in the second jar on standing? Can you account for the difference in the two results?

3. What change occurs in the bowl of water and oil when you add the detergent? Does the surface change? Why?

Discussion

1. What is an emulsion?

2. What kind of emulsion was formed in the water-oil mixtures?

19

3. What was the function of the liquid detergent on the water and oil mixture in the bowl?

4. What is the function of an emulsifying agent?

5. What agent performs this emulsification in digestion and absorption of fats in the body and how does it act?

Individual or Group Project: Food Fat Products

Materials and setting Paper and pencil for note taking, newspapers and magazines, television set, community food market.

Procedure
1. Visit the selected community market and survey the fats and fat related foods. Read the labels carefully.
2. Look for fat-related terms used on labels, such as "P/S ratio," "imitation," "hydrogenated," "fortified," "hardened," "saturated," "polyunsaturated."
3. Include the following types of foods in your survey: shortenings, margarines, oils, frozen desserts, whipped toppings, cream substitutes or nondairy creamers, milks, egg and cheese foods, egg substitutes, special low-fat cheeses.

Results
1. Compare the labels on the food products. Record the descriptive terms that you located and describe the product involved. What does each term mean? How has the product been processed?

2. Compare the labels on various margarines carefully. The listed ingredients on products must be given in the order of amount or predominance of that ingredient in the product. What product, therefore, would you select as being the most unsaturated margarine? Why?

3. How is margarine like butter? How does it differ from butter?

4.	How are shortening and margarine produced?

5.	What difference did you find in the frozen desserts?

6.	How many different milks did you find? How do they differ?

7.	Compare dairy creamers in both powder and liquid form. How do they differ from cream?

8.	Compare the results of your market survey with any television, newspaper, or magazine advertisements for fats and fat-related food products. What information did you find in the advertisement? What is your evaluation of these ads?

Discussion
1.	Describe the chemical concept of saturation as applied to the structure and form of fats. What physical characteristics result?

2.	What is the significance to human health of the degree of fat saturation in foods?

Situational Problem
	Refer again to the situation of Dick Smith (p 11), the young man with diabetes. After he is feeling better, he continues his studying while he eats his snack of a peanut butter and butter sandwich and a glass of milk.

1.	What are the fat sources of energy in Dick's snack?

2. What changes must his body make in these sources to get them into a form the cells can use to burn for energy?

3. What important relationship do carbohydrate and fat have in the final production of energy in the body?

4. If Dick did not take his insulin to provide the necessary control agent for metabolizing the carbohydrate, what would happen to him as a result of improper handling of fat and the resulting accumulation of ketones?

Individual Diet Analysis

Record in detail your food intake for a day, including meals and snack items. Use the Daily Food Intake box on p 292 to list your day's food and check each of the fat items. Trace what happens to them in your body.

Current Nutritional Issues

Read carefully the *Issues and Answers* article, "The Dietary Fat and Cholesterol Controversy" (*Essentials of Nutrition and Diet Therapy*, ed 6, p 60; *Nutrition and Diet Therapy*, ed 7, p 82). Consider these inquiry questions:

1. What current evidence do we have of a diet-heart disease link?

2. Do you think lipid-screening is important for members of high-risk families with strong history of coronary heart disease and hypertension? (Refer also to Chapter 20.)

3. Why do you think Americans over the past few decades developed food habits of increased fat intake? Why is it difficult to reduce these habits of fat intake? Have you or any of your family or friends changed habits of fat use recently? Why did you make these diet habit changes?

4.   Consider the development of U.S. dietary guides issued for health promotion (See Chapter 1). What evidence do you see in food markets that the food-processing industry is responding to these public concerns about dietary fat and cholesterol? Give examples from food product labels.

Chapter 4
PROTEINS

Chapter Focus

Individual human beings are unique. We have specific tissue proteins that are made by specific building units—amino acids—arranged in specific patterns under specific genetic control. These required amino acids are supplied by our food proteins to constantly build and maintain our bodies.

Summary-Review Quiz

Fill in the blanks below with the appropriate number and word(s) from the list following each section. Each numbered word is used; some may be used more than once. When you've completed all the sections, check your answers for each blank against the test key. Correct any mistakes and then review the entire chapter summary.

1. Protein, like carbohydrate and fat, is composed of the basic chemical elements: _____, _____, and _____. Unlike carbohydrate and fat, however, it also contains _____, the key element for all living beings on this planet. Some proteins may also include other elements such as _____.

2. Proteins are very _____ structures, put together by a _____ plan just for that protein. Thus the primary function of protein is that of _____. Proteins are _____ of high _____. Their unit building blocks are the _____.

3. Diets of many people in the underdeveloped countries of the world, as well as in poverty areas of our own country, lack _____. Because protein is basic to life, such deficiency is a major _____. In adequately fed populations, however, protein contributes about 12% to 20% of the total _____ of the diet.

1. nitrogen	6. complex compounds	11. particular
2. specific	7. good quality protein	12. carbon
3. molecular weight	8. hydrogen	13. building tissue
4. oxygen	9. world health problem	14. sulfur
5. kilocalories	10. amino acids	

4. Pure protein food does not occur naturally, with one exception: _____. Animal food proteins also contain _____. Plant food proteins also contain _____.

5. Protein building units that the body cannot manufacture are called _____.
Therefore they are _____ in the diet. Protein foods that contain all of these
_____ in sufficient amounts have high nutritive value. Such protein foods are
called _____ and are found only in _____ sources. Of these, the one
with the highest nutritive value is _____. The others are _____,
including seafood, and the dairy products _____ and _____. Protein
foods that lack sufficient amounts of one or more necessary building units are called
_____ and come from _____ sources, such as _____,
_____, nuts, and _____.

1. incomplete proteins
2. egg
3. animal
4. necessary
5. legumes

6. fat
7. milk
8. essential amino acids
9. cheese
10. complete proteins

11. plant
12. egg white albumin
13. seeds
14. meat
15. carbohydrate
16. grains

6. The structural building blocks of proteins, the _____, have a dual chemical
structure containing both an _____ factor and a _____ factor. This dual
structure enables _____ to join in a _____ to form long chains called
_____. This long coiled chain, then, is the specific protein.
7. Because proteins are complex compounds, food proteins require a series of
_____ for digestion. This breakdown of protein is begun in the _____
by the _____ enzyme, _____. It is continued in the _____ by
the _____ enzymes: trypsin, chymotrypsin, and carboxypeptidase. Also the
_____ enzyme, aminopeptidase, splits off the _____ (nitrogen-
containing) end of the peptide chain, and dipeptidase finally completes the separation of
the chain fragment dipeptides to produce _____. These are the end products of
protein digestion. These basic units of protein structure are then absorbed through the
wall of the small intestine with the aid of _____ as a carrier and carried to the
cells for their primary _____ function.

1. pepsin
2. free amino acids
3. peptide linkage
4. pancreatic
5. acid

6. small intestine
7. enzymes
8. tissue-building
9. gastric
10. amino acids

11. pyridoxine (vitamin B_6)
12. amino
13. polypeptides
14. intestinal
15. stomach
16. base

8. In the cells, according to metabolic needs, specific proteins are always being _____ and _____ and rebuilt in a constant balance to maintain health. The many built-in body controls that govern this overall equilibrium are called _____. They are life-sustaining. This protein turnover is greatest in _____ tissues, such as the intestinal mucosa, liver, pancreas, kidney, and blood plasma. Little protein turnover occurs in _____ tissue or other skeletal structures.

9. To ensure a constant supply of needed amino acids, the tissues maintain a _____ of reserve amino acids. This reserve comes from both _____ and _____ sources.

10. The body's overall protein balance is measured in terms of _____. This refers to the relation of total _____ in food to the total _____ in body excretions or losses. When the nitrogen or protein losses exceed the nitrogen or protein intake, a state of _____ exists. Such a state occurs, for example, in _____ or long-term illness or following _____. A normal state of _____ occurs in periods of _____ and during pregnancy.

1. nitrogen balance	6. nitrogen output	11. metabolically active
2. starvation	7. broken down	12. surgery
3. childhood growth	8. negative nitrogen balance	13. nitrogen intake
4. metabolic pool	9. body tissue	14. built
5. homeostatic mechanisms	10. positive nitrogen balance	15. dietary
		16. collagenous

11. The process of building tissue through the synthesis of new proteins is called _____. This specific process is carried out under the control of a specific pattern, or "blueprint," which is set by the _____ in the cell nucleus. This pattern is transferred to the cell-building sites, the _____. Here the specific amino acids are guided into place and joined together to build the _____. Control agents that stimulate and regulate these vital tissue-building activities are the _____ and _____.

12. The process of breaking down tissue protein and releasing its structural units, the _____, is called _____. These structural units are then available for new protein synthesis. If they are not used in building, they may be broken down to produce: (1) the _____ that may be excreted in the urine or used in building another _____ and (2) the remaining _____ carbon residue. This residue may be converted to carbohydrate or fat and used for _____, or it may be used in building still another _____.

1. specific proteins	6. energy	11. nitrogen-containing part
2. non-nitrogen	7. catabolism	12. ribosomes
3. deoxyribonucleic acid (DNA)	8. amino acid	
4. amino acids	9. anabolism	
5. cell enzymes	10. hormones	

13. Individual requirements for _____ are determined by the size of the individual, the state of growth and health, and the _____ in the diet. For example, _____ protein is needed during pregnancy and lactation, in the rapid growth period during _____, in debilitating disease, and in _____ after injury or _____.

14. Protein requirements ultimately are based mainly on the _____ of dietary protein. This _____ depends on the amount of the _____ present in the food. A _____ diet, for example, may be lacking in these _____ and would need to be planned carefully around complementary _____ to achieve the necessary ratio and balance of these necessary structural units.

15. The RDA standards of the _____ for protein are not meant to serve as rigid _____ protein requirements but as flexible recommended guidelines for the health of _____ with a variety of individual protein needs. Thus they should be _____ as a point of reference for _____ protein needs.

1. increased	6. wound healing	11. National Research Council
2. plant proteins	7. adapted	12. adolescence
3. vegetarian	8. quality	13. population groups
4. quality of protein	9. surgery	14. essential amino acids
5. individual	10. protein	

Discussion Questions

1. What reasons can you give for the increased demands for protein during pregnancy? Would this increase also apply during the following lactation period? Why?

2. What is meant by the "dual nature" of amino acid structure? What can the amino acids do as the result of this significant structure?

3. Why is such an involved series of digestive enzymes necessary to handle protein food?

4. For a person suffering from extensive burns, a great deal of extra protein is required. Why would this be vital to recovery?

5. What is meant by the term *nutritive value* as applied to protein foods? How do complete and incomplete proteins differ?

6. Considering the wide variety of tissues and cells in the human body, how is the synthesis of a *specific* tissue protein controlled?

Self-Test Questions

True-False
Circle the "T" if a statement is true and write a brief rationale for its accuracy. If it is false, circle the "F" and write the correct statement.

T F 1. Complete protein of high biologic value are found in whole grains, dried beans and peas, and nuts.

T F 2. The primary function of dietary protein is to supply the necessary amino acids to build and repair body tissue.

T F 3. Proteins provide a main source of body heat and muscle energy.

T F 4. Proteins play a large role in the resistance of the body to disease.

T F 5. In the average American diet, protein foods comprise 5% to 7% of the total caloric intake.

T F 6. Because they are smaller, children need less protein per unit of body weight than adults require.

T F 7. In old age the protein requirement decreases because of lessened physical activity.

T F	8.	The structure of an individual person is influenced by the kind and amount of protein in the diet.
T F	9.	Throughout much of the world the shortage of protein is a paramount health problem.
T F	10.	The healthy adult is in a state of nitrogen balance.
T F	11.	Positive nitrogen balance exists during the ages of rapid growth, such as in early childhood and during puberty.
T F	12.	When a negative nitrogen balance exists, the person is less able to resist infections and general health deteriorates.
T F	13.	Cheese has an equal protein value to that of meat because of its high biologic value.
T F	14.	Wheat and rice are complete protein foods of high biologic value.
T F	15.	The protein in egg has a higher biologic value than the value of protein in meat.

Multiple Choice

Circle the letter in front of the correct answer. Then check your answers by the test key (p 247). Now compare all the possible answers for each item and write the following brief statements: (1) rationale for the correct answer and (2) why each one of the other responses is incorrect.

1. Twenty-two amino acids are involved in total body metabolism, building and rebuilding various tissues. Of these, 9 are termed *essential* amino acids. This means that:
   a. the body cannot synthesize these 9 amino acids and hence must obtain them in the diet
   b. these 9 amino acids are essential in body processes, and the remaining 13 are not
   c. these 9 amino acids can be made by the body because they are essential to life
   d. after synthesizing these 9 amino acids, the body uses them in key processes essential for growth

2. A complete food protein of high nutritive value would be one that contains:
   a. all 22 of the amino acids in sufficient quantity to meet human requirements
   b. the 9 essential amino acids in any proportion, since the body can always fill in the difference needed
   c. all of the 22 amino acids from which the body can make additional amounts of the 9 essential amino acids needed
   d. all 9 of the essential amino acids in correct proportion to meet human needs

3. Which one of the following statements correctly describes the digestive processes by which food protein is changed into basic structural materials, amino acids for building and maintaining tissue?
   a. Since protein is a relatively simple structure, its digestive breakdown occurs easily.

29

    b.   Proteins are complex structure of high molecular weight, requiring a series of strong enzymes to digest them.
    c.   The initial enzymes in the protein-splitting system are strongly active substances, first secreted for immediate effectiveness.
    d.   The stomach acid (HCl) has no relation to the initial digestion of protein.
4. The end products of protein digestion, the amino acids, are absorbed from the small intestine by the process of:
    a.   simple diffusion because of their small size
    b.   active transport with the aid of vitamin B_6 in its active form
    c.   osmosis because of their greater concentration in the intestinal lumen
    d.   filtration according to the osmotic pressure direction
5. In each cell a constant balance is maintained between the building up an breaking down of tissue protein. In this way a state of dynamic equilibrium is maintained throughout the body. This state is called:
    a.   anabolism
    b.   catabolism
    c.   energy balance
    d.   homeostasis

Learning Activities

Situational Problem
    A neighbor of yours is 20 years old and has just discovered that she is pregnant with her first child. She says that she and her husband are "vegetarians." She asks your advice about her diet.
1. What growth material is one of her basic nutritional needs during her pregnancy?

2. What further information would you want about her diet habits to help her meet this need?

3. What foods would you try first to have her use in increased amounts? Why?

4. If you learned that she is a true vegetarian (vegan) using only plant foods, how would you help her get enough growth materials.

5. Why would adequate carbohydrate foods also be important in her prenatal diet?

Individual Diet Analysis

Record in detail your food intake for a day, including all meal and snack items. Use the Daily Food Intake box on p. 293 to list your day's food and check each item containing protein. Calculate your total protein intake and the total caloric value of your diet, using the food value tables in the appendix of your text.

1. What percentage of your total kcalories is contributed by protein?

2. What is your general protein requirement according to your weight and age?

3. Compare your calculated protein intake with the RDA standard. Is your protein intake adequate, deficient, or excessive?

Current Nutritional Issues

Read carefully the *Issues and Answers* article "Vegetarian Food Patterns: Harm or Health?" (*Essentials of Nutrition and Diet Therapy*, ed 6, p 75); ("The Vegetarian Revolution," *Nutrition and Diet Therapy*, ed 7, p 104). Consider these inquiry questions:

1. In evaluating vegetarian diets, why is it important to distinguish among the various forms? What forms are dangerous to health?

2. What are some of the values of a vegetarian diet? What forms of vegetarianism would support positive health?

3. Are nutrient supplements needed by a person on a vegetarian diet? Why or why not?

4. What dietary counsel would you provide for a person on a vegetarian diet who is a pregnant woman? A young child? An overweight adult?

Chapter 5
DIGESTION, ABSORPTION, AND METABOLISM

Chapter Focus

The continuous integrated processes of digestion, absorption, and metabolism change the food we eat into multiple interactive nutrients and intermediate compounds that are necessary to sustain human life. These constant chemical changes and balances provide the framework and flesh of nutritional science.

Summary-Review Quiz

Fill in the blanks below with the appropriate number and word(s) from the list following each section. Each numbered word is used; some may be used more than once. When you've completed all the sections, check your answers for each blank against the test key. Correct any mistakes and then review the entire chapter summary.

1.   Many changes by which food is prepared for use by the _____ to sustain life are brought about by the successive processes of _____, _____, and _____. But these processes make up one continuous, interrelated whole. This basic concept of wholeness, or _____, is a fundamental physiologic truth. Food components, the _____, travel together through the successive parts of the _____ and into the _____, the functional units of life.

2.   This intricate and complex biochemical and physiologic life system is necessary because humans are the most highly developed creates and their _____ as it exists naturally cannot meet _____ life needs. Its components must be _____, _____, and _____ to fulfill specific life requirements. This is the integrated physiochemical picture of human nutrition.

1. metabolism
2. food
3. digestion
4. broken apart
5. biochemical

6. nutrients
7. absorption
8. body integrity
9. regrouped
10. body cells

11. gastrointestinal system
12. simplified

3.   The initial preparation of food for use by the body is achieved by the process of _____. The two basic types of actions involved are _____ and _____.

4.   A system of interrelated _____ and _____ moves the food mass along the gastrointestinal tract at a rate and in a form that allows chemical _____ and _____ of the nutrients in the food to take place.   Alternating muscle contractions and relaxations force the food mass forward by a process called _____.   Special _____ form valves at key points to regulate progressive passage of the contents--the _____, _____, and _____ valves. A specific interrelated _____ extends the length of the system and controls all its coordinated actions.

1. sphincter muscles	6. absorption	11. peristalsis
2. network of nerves	7. anal	12. mechanical activities
3. muscles	8. chemical reactions	
4. pyloric	9. ileocecal	
5. nerves	10. digestion	

5.   The food components are digested chemically by a system of _____. These chemical catalysts are aided by three other types of secretions: _____ to maintain the required pH, _____ to aid passage of the food mass, and _____ to provide a solution base and transport medium.   These materials are secreted by special cells of the mucosal tissue of the gastrointestinal tract under the stimulus of local food pressure as well as _____ and _____.

6.   In the mouth, _____ of the food breaks it up into smaller pieces and mixes it into a mass that can be swallowed and carried down the _____ into the _____.   A _____ at this point relaxes to allow the food to enter but closes again to prevent _____.

7.   Sometimes a problem develops here in the form of a _____, an outpouching of the upper stomach wall into the thorax, which harbors food and slows its normal passage at this point.

1. water and electrolytes	6. specific hormones	11. esophagus
2. mastication	7. mucus	12. sensory nerves
3. stomach	8. constrictor muscle	
4. HCl and buffer ions	9. specific enzymes	
5. regurgitation	10. hiatal hernia	

8.   Up to now little chemical change has occurred. In the mouth, _____ glands secrete _____, an enzyme specific for _____, but food usually leaves the mouth too fast for this enzyme to act in any large measure.

9.   In the stomach a churning sort of _____ mixes the food with gastric juices and mucus to reduce it to a semifluid _____.   At the juncture of the stomach and the small intestine, the _____ releases the _____ semiliquid food mass slowly, so that it can be buffered by the _____ intestinal secretions.

10.   The gastric juices contain hydrochloric acid, mucus, and _____, of which the main one is _____, to begin the digestion of protein. A small amount of _____ is produced to act on butterfat, but this is a minor activity. In infancy and childhood an enzyme called _____ is also present to aid in the coagulation of milk.

1. ptyalin
2. muscle action
3. enzymes
4. rennin
5. acid
6. gastric lipase
7. pyloric valve
8. pepsin
9. alkaline
10. salivary
11. chyme
12. starch

11.   Up to this point, digestion has been mainly _____, producing a semifluid _____. The major _____ digestion and nutrient _____ occurs in the _____, aided by finely coordinated layers of _____ and absorbing structures.

12.   This _____ digestion in the small intestine is accomplished by three main types of secretions: (1) large amounts of protective _____ from intestinal glands in the first section of the duodenum, (2) _____, an emulsifying agent for fats secreted by the _____ and stored in the _____, and (3) a large number of _____ secreted by the pancreas and the intestine. Thus the small intestine, together with its three accessory organs, the _____, _____, and _____, completes the _____ breakdown of the nutrients, making them now ready for absorption.

1. mucus
2. muscles
3. pancreas
4. chyme
5. absorption
6. gallbladder
7. chemical
8. liver
9. mechanical
10. bile
11. specific enzymes
12. small intestine

13.   The end products of nutrient digestion include : (1) carbohydrates: the simple sugars (monosaccharides), _____, _____, and _____; (2) from fats: _____, _____, and _____; and (3) from proteins: _____. Also released are vitamins and minerals.

14.   Three basic structures of the intestinal mucosa greatly increase its absorbing surface. In successively smaller size, these structures are the _____, _____, and _____.

15.   Each intestinal villus contains both _____ and _____ vessels to carry these nutrient products into the portal circulation. Water-soluble _____ and _____ products can go directly into the portal blood system. However, most fat products are not water-soluble and must travel the _____ route first for preparation before finally reaching the portal circulation.

1. fatty acids
2. glycerol
3. microvilli
4. lymph
5. galactose

6. protein
7. blood
8. mucosal folds
9. fructose
10. amino acids

11. glucose
12. glycerides
13. carbohydrate
14. villi

16.   In the large intestine, the final section of the gastrointestinal tract, the main task left is _____ . Here also, intestinal absorption of _____ provides the major means of controlling their amounts in the body. Bacteria in the colon synthesize some of the _____, which are then absorbed to help meet daily needs. Undigested _____ contributes bulk to form and eliminate the _____.

17.   The various absorbed nutrients, now in the form of _____, _____, and _____, are carried to the cells for cell metabolism. The overall final processes of cell metabolism involve all the complex, interrelated chemical changes that _____ and _____.

1. refined fuels
2. build tissue
3. feces
4. minerals

5. metabolic control agents
6. dietary fiber
7. water absorption
8. provide energy

9. building units
10. vitamins

Discussion Questions

1.   How do the interrelated concepts of change and balance relate to the overall process of digestion-absorption-metabolism? Why is this intricate system necessary?

2.   How do the mechanical and chemical aspects of digestion support one another in a common goal? How are these two aspects of digestion controlled?

3. What is an enzyme? How does it work? What is meant by the *specificity* of enzyme action?

4. Hydrochloric acid is irritating and destructive to gastric tissue, and large amounts of mucus have to be secreted to protect the stomach lining. If this is true, why must the hydrochloric acid be produced at all? Why is it necessary in digestion? What does it do?

5. How is the intestinal mucosa structured to facilitate absorption? How large an absorbing surface do these unique structures provide?

6. Why are many of the mechanisms for absorbing nutrients called *pumps*?

7. The major absorption of nutrients takes place in the small intestine. What then remains as the task of the large intestine?

Self-Test Questions

<u>True-False</u>
    Circle the "T" if a statement is true and write a brief rationale for its accuracy. If it is false, circle the "F" and write the correct statement.

T F 1. The ileocecal valve controls the release of acid gastric contents into the duodenum.
T F 2. The digestive products of a large meal are difficult to absorb because the overall area of the intestinal absorbing surface is relatively small.
T F 3. Some enzymes must be activated by hydrochloric acid or other enzymes before they can act.
T F 4. Bile is a specific enzyme for fats.
T F 5. One enzyme may work on more than one nutrient.
T F 6. The "gastrointestinal circulation" provides a constant supply of water and electrolytes to carry the digestive substances being produced.

T F 7. Secretions from the gastrointestinal accessory organs, the gallbladder and pancreas, mix with gastric secretions to aid digestion.

T F 8. Bile is released from the gallbladder in response to the cholecystokinin hormone stimulus.

Multiple Choice

Circle the letter in front of the correct answer. Then check your answers by the test key (p 248). Now compare all the possible answers for each item and write the following brief statements: (1) rationale for the correct answer and (2) why each one of the other responses is incorrect.

1. During digestion the food mass is moved forward by periodic rhythmic muscle action called:
   a. sphincter contraction
   b. contractile ring motion
   c. tonic waves
   d. peristalsis

2. Gastrointestinal secretory action is triggered by:
   (1) hormones
   (2) enzymes
   (3) nerve network
   (4) sensory stimuli
   a. 1 and 2
   b. 2 and 4
   c. 1, 3, and 4
   d. 2 and 3

3. Mucus is an important gastrointestinal secretion because it:
   a. causes chemical changes in some substances to prepare them for enzyme action
   b. helps create the proper degree of acidity for enzymes to act
   c. lubricates and protects the gastrointestinal lining
   d. helps to emulsify fats

4. The pyloric valve controls:
   a. regurgitation of swallowed food materials
   b. release of gastric contents into the duodenum
   c. passage of food mass from small intestine to large intestine
   d. elimination of feces

5. Pepsin is:
   a. produced in the small intestine to act on protein
   b. a gastric enzyme that acts on protein
   c. produced in the pancreas to act on fat
   d. produced in the small intestine to act on fats

6. Which of the following food combinations remains longest in the stomach?
    a. egg and a slice of toast with jelly
    b. a glass of nonfat milk with cookies
    c. sliced banana over dry cereal with nonfat milk
    d. a roast beef sandwich on buttered bread
7. Bile is an important secretion that is:
    a. produced by the gallbladder
    b. stored in the liver
    c. an aid to protein digestion
    d. an emulsifier for fats
8. The enterohepatic circulation of bile provides a mechanism for:
    a. eliminating the major portion of the large amounts of bile produced daily by the body
    b. reabsorbing most of the bile used daily in fat digestion and absorption so that very little is lost
    c. producing more bile as needed to replace losses
    d. breaking down bile after it is used so that an excessive accumulation is prevented
9. The route of fat absorption is:
    a. the lymphatic system via the villi lacteals
    b. directly into the portal circulation
    c. with the aid of bile directly into the villi blood capillaries
    d. with the aid of protein directly into the portal circulation as lipoproteins
10. The important fat-clearing blood factor that handles large fat loads following a meal is:
    a. gastric lipase
    b. pancreatic lipase
    c. enteric lipase
    d. lipoprotein lipase

Learning Activities

Individual Experiment: Gastric Emptying Time and the Satiety of Food
Materials Fruit, fruit juice, white bread, jelly, butter or margarine, eggs, tea, sugar, coffee, cream.
Procedure On each morning of 3 successive days eat the following breakfasts and record the time that you first felt hungry after each one:
Day 1: Breakfast A
    All fruit breakfast. Eat several fruits and fruit juices only.
Day 2: Breakfast B
    Eat only fruit juice, one or two slices of white toast with jelly, and hot tea with sugar.

Day 3: Breakfast C

Eat only one or two slices of toast with a generous amount of butter or margarine, two eggs scrambled in melted butter or margarine, and coffee with cream and sugar if desired.

<u>Results</u>   Record your response to each breakfast:

1.   Which food combination satisfied you for the longest period of time?

2.   Which food combination left you hungry sooner?

<u>Discussion</u>

1.   What type breakfast—A, B, or C—provided the slowest gastric emptying time? The fastest? Why?

2.   In what order do nutrients leave the stomach? Why?

3.   What does the word *satiety* mean? How does it apply to your findings here?

<u>Group Experiment: Effect of Hydrochloric Acid on Tissue</u>

<u>Materials</u>   Hydrochloric acid, a strip of bacon, and a piece of cotton material.

<u>Procedure</u>

1.   Pour hydrochloric acid into a jar and dilute with a little water.
2.   Cut bacon into pieces and add to the acid solution. Observe results.
3.   Drop some undiluted hydrochloric acid on the piece of cloth. Observe results.

<u>Results</u>

1.   What was the appearance of the bacon during the first few moments after putting it in the acid solution?

2.   What was the appearance of the bacon after a 1- or 2-hour interval of time had passed?

3.   What happened on the spot of cloth where the hydrochloric acid was placed?

Discussion

1.   What action does hydrochloric acid have on tissue?

2.   How is this action prevented in human digestion?

3.   What kind of substance is the cotton cloth? What is the effect of hydrochloric acid on cotton? Why does this happen?

Current Nutrition Issues

Read carefully the *Issues and Answers* article "Lactose Intolerance: Common Problem Worldwide" (*Essentials of Nutrition and Diet Therapy*, ed 6, p 33; *Nutrition and Diet Therapy*, ed 7, p 41). Consider these inquiry questions:

1.   Why do you think relief agencies often include dry milk in their food shipments to famine-stricken areas of the world?

2.   Why does a majority of the world's population have an intolerance for milk?

3. Why would fermented milk products be better tolerated? Why can't they be used instead in such relief programs?

4. What is a solution to this problem, one that would allow such persons the nutritional benefits of milk?

Chapter 6
ENERGY BALANCE AND WEIGHT MANAGEMENT

Chapter Focus

Energy balance reflects the human energy system's actions to take in energy as food fuel, then change and transform it to yield both free and potential energy for our life-sustaining body work. This energy is measured in kilocalories.

Despite an obsession with thinness and weight loss, as a people Americans are getting heavier, largely due to our growing technology and its sedentary society. The traditional medical (or illness) model of obesity is being reevaluated. Today a more realistic positive health model of weight and fitness management combines good food habits with increased physical activity and self-esteem.

Summary-Review Quiz

Fill in the blanks below with the appropriate number and word(s) from the list following each section. Each numbered word or word group is used; some may be used more than once. When you have completed all the sections, check your answers for each blank by the test key (Appendix, p 249). Correct any mistakes and then review the entire chapter summary.

Energy Balance
1.   The human energy system is based on constant _____ in the basic fuels, _____ and _____, and the back-up energy nutrient, _____, to release energy for the body's _____. Since this _____ produces heat, human energy is measured in terms of heat equivalents called _____. In human nutrition this term refers to a _____, which is the amount of heat required to raise 1 _____ of water 1° C.
2.   The _____ of various foods are calculated according to the fuel factors of their component nutrients. For example, 1 g of carbohydrate yields _____, 1 g of fat yields _____, and 1 g of protein yields _____. The international unit of measure for energy is the _____. With this system of measure, 4.184 kilojoules equals 1 _____.

1. kilocalorie values	5. calories	9. 9 kilocalories
2. 4 kilocalories	6. kilogram	10. kilocalorie
3. joule	7. carbohydrate	11. fat
4. protein	8. work	12. chemical changes

43

3.   When we eat food, we are not really _____ energy from it. We are _____ the stored _____ energy in the food by _____ it to other forms of energy, such as _____, _____, _____, and _____ energy. These are then _____ throughout the system. The ultimate source of all energy in our system is the _____. With the benefit of this energy source, plants use the raw materials _____ and _____ to produce fuel foods. The body then converts these foods into the refined fuel units _____ and _____, burning them to release energy.

1. changing	6. chemical	11. producing
2. sun	7. cycled	12. glucose
3. electrical	8. fatty acids	13. thermal
4. transforming	9. potential	14. carbon dioxide
5. water	10. mechanical	

4.   The main means of the control necessary in the human energy system is _____. This may be in the form of covalent bonds, such as those holding together the core _____ atoms of organic compounds. Easily broken bonds that help form many new compounds are those formed by _____. Others include _____ bonds, which are _____ bonds used to _____ energy as it is produced, so that it can be released as needed. A main example of the latter form is _____.

5.   The nature and rate of the many chemical reactions in the cells that form the human energy system are controlled by _____, each of which is a specific _____ compound. Each one works on its _____, locking together and forming new metabolic products. Some reactions also require a _____ partner, many of which involve _____ and _____. Other specific metabolic reactions are regulated by _____, which act as chemical messengers to trigger or control specific enzyme actions.

1. high energy	6. vitamins	11. hydrogen
2. enzymes	7. phosphate	12. minerals
3. adenosine triphosphate (ATP)	8. coenzyme	13. trap and store
4. specific substrate	9. chemical bonding	14. protein
5. carbon	10. hormones	

6.   Metabolic reactions may build up more complex substances from simpler ones, a process called _____. Other reactions may break down complex substances to simpler ones, a process called _____. These two types of processes are constantly going on to maintain the body in a state of _____, or equilibrium.

7.   Stored forms of body energy are _____, _____, and _____. Of these, the _____ stores are smallest, providing only a 12- to 48-hour reserve. The _____ stores in the form of _____ are almost unlimited depending on individual body size and composition.

8.   The energy needed to carry on the body's internal work at rest is called its _____ requirement. The measure of energy required by the activities of resting tissue is called the _____. The major factor influencing this measure is _____, to which factors such as age and _____ relate. Other influencing factors include _____, _____, and _____. These _____ requirements average about _____ per _____ of body weight per _____.

1. glycogen	7. 1 kilocalorie	13. basal metabolic rate
2. fat	8. lean body mass	14. climate
3. basal energy	9. dynamic balance	15. anabolism
4. growth	10. fever and disease	16. hour
5. catabolism	11. basal metabolic	17. sex
6. adipose tissue	12. kilogram	18. muscle mass

9.   The remaining energy requirement is added by _____, mainly in the form of muscle work. Some additional energy is required for _____ and _____ food and its nutrients. This stimulating effect of food is called the _____, and accounts for about _____ of the total metabolic needs. A heightened _____ state also requires added energy. Few if any additional kilocalories are required for _____.

10.   A person's _____ is a general indicator of the state of _____ between _____ and energy used in the _____ and _____ needs.

1. thermic effect of food	5. basal	9. 10% to 15%
2. digesting	6. emotional	10. mental effort
3. weight	7. food	11. absorbing
4. physical activities	8. activity	12. energy balance

Weight Management

1.   Obesity is a clinical term for _____ over 20% of _____. It is associated as a _____ with (1) _____ and (2) _____, and thus indirectly with (3) _____ disease. About _____ of the American population is on some sort of _____ diet and a _____ is widespread.

2.   Efforts to deal with this situation are frustrating, largely because obesity and _____ are difficult to define by the usual standard _____. The critical factor is _____, how much weight comes from fat and how much from _____.

1. risk factor	6. height-weight tables	11. excess body weight
2. body composition	7. ideal weight	12. weight reduction
3. 25%	8. cardiovascular	13. diabetes mellitus
4. hypertension	9. fear of fatness	
5. overweight	10. lean body mass	

3. Questions have been raised about standard _____ as a measure of _____ weight. Problems exist with the _____ on which these standards are based and how _____ they may be of our _____. Health risks lie with _____ as well as with _____ ones. Excessive _____ as well as excessive _____ is to be avoided. Many health problems attributed to _____ are unfounded. The facts of _____ and need for _____ make setting an _____ standard a problem. For example, for reproductive health, women require about _____.

1. total population
2. individual variation
3. very fat
4. desirable
5. moderate overweight

6. ideal weight
7. representative
8. underweight
9. body fat
10. life insurance data

11. 20% body fat
12. very thin persons
13. height-weight tables
14. overweight

4. The basic physical laws of _____ account for obesity. This means the _____ in excess of _____ produces obesity. However, the level of this _____ varies with individual _____.

5. Some physiological causes of obesity may relate to _____ in early childhood years, decreased _____ during the elementary school years, adolescent _____ differences in body composition, and _____ adjustments in adulthood between habitual food intake and lessened _____. Two theories have developed to account for these obesity problems: (1) the _____ of excess fat cells from childhood due to _____ and _____ and (2) the _____ of an internal mechanism regulating the amount of _____.

1. overfeeding
2. energy balance
3. caloric balance
4. sex
5. genetics

6. caloric intake
7. body fat
8. metabolic efficiency
9. set-point theory
10. energy exchange

11. physical activity
12. eating patterns
13. fat cell theory
14. caloric expenditure

6. Social factors such as _____ and cultural factors of _____ and _____ also influence obesity.

7. Other _____ associated with obesity are also experienced as well by many _____ and _____ persons. Various _____ factors such as boredom, lonliness, or _____ may cause _____ and weight _____ or _____ and weight _____.

1. psychologic factors
2. reduced food intake
3. meal pattern
4. rejection

5. thin
6. gain
7. holiday feasting
8. stress

9. overeating
10. loss
11. class values
12. average weight

46

8. Successful approaches to weight management are based on several factors. First, there must be a strong personal _____ and decision to achieve and maintain a healthy weight. Second, some type of _____ must be provided to carry out the decision in a wise continuing program. Third, there must be a sound _____ based on the reduction of excess _____ and adapted realistically to the _____. Fourth, some kind of _____ must be worked out to help continue the _____ and _____ the healthy weight once it is achieved. The program must meet _____ and provide guidance for behavioral changes in _____ habits, _____ training, and development of _____.

1. personal food plan	5. support	9. motivation
2. food and exercise	6. maintain	10. follow-up plan
3. individual life situation	7. food habit changes	11. personal needs
4. personal interest areas	8. relaxation	12. kilocalories

9. Certain characteristics are therefore essential in a sound food plan for weight management. Individual goals must be _____ in terms of weight loss desired and rate of loss. Total _____ in the diet must supply all needed _____. The food plan must be _____ and personally acceptable, so as to help with _____ of eating habits. When the weight goal is reached, the _____ must be readjusted to _____ the weight at the healthy individually natural level.

10. The best approach, however, to the problem of _____ and weight management would seem to be _____. Attention to (1) early _____ of young children, (2) changes in the value placed on _____ foods, high-density foods rich in _____, and (3) early _____ to help avoid _____ before it becomes a problem.

1. energy balance	6. kilocalories	11. prevention
2. feeding practices	7. culturally	12. nutrients
3. permanent reeducation	8. maintain	13. high-caloric
4. fat and suagr	9. nutrition education	14. lowered
5. obesity	10. realistic	

Discussion Questions

1.   Describe the process by which plants produce energy.

2.   What is the difference between potential energy and free energy?

47

3.   How is energy in the human energy system measured?

4.   How is "energy production" controlled in the human body? Is "energy production" actually a correct term to use in describing the body's energy system? Support your answer.

5.   What does a BMR test measure? What does REE mean? How does it compare with BMR?

6.   Thyroid function tests are frequently used to indicate BMR. What are some of these indirect tests?

7.   Why is there a problem in defining "ideal" weight?

8.   Select any current fad reducing diet and evaluate it in terms of the essentrial characteristics of a sound diet for weight management.

9.   Since prevention is the wisest approach to the problem of obesity, suggest ways that this might be accomplished in each of the following stages of the life cycle: (1) infancy, (2) toddler period, (3) preschool years, (4) elementary school years, (5) adolescence, and (6) adulthood.

10. What health problems may be associated with obesity? Why?

Self-Test Questions

True-False
        Circle the "T" if a statement is true and write a brief rationale for its accuracy. If it is false, circle the "F" and write the correct statement.

T F   1.   Starvation and malnutrition states increase the body's basal metabolic rate.
T F   2.   Pregnancy raises the BMR more than does subsequent lactation.
T F   3.   Disease usually lowers the BMR.
T F   4.   Glycogen stores provide a long-lasting energy reserve.
T F   5.   The process of catabolism creates new, more complex, metabolic products.
T F   6.   An enzyme may control several different metabolic reactions.
T F   7.   Hydrogen bonds are high-energy bonds.
T F   8.   Electrical energy is used in brain and nerve activity.
T F   9.   The end products of energy-yielding body metabolism are carbon dioxide and water.
T F   10.   Kilocalories are nutrients in food.
T F   11.   Appetite is an instinctive response to specific foods.
T F   12.   Satiety is a sense of satisfaction after eating, with a lack of desire to eat more.
T F   13.   Hunger is a learned physiologic habit response to food.
T F   14.   Developmental childhood obesity results from genetics and eating patterns and produces an excess ratio of fat to lean tissue.
T F   15.   Increasing the amount of energy expended for physical activity is an important aspect of weight management.
T F   16.   During adolescence the boy usually has the higher deposit of subcutaneous fat tissue than the girl.
T F   17.   The energy value of a reasonable weight reduction diet usually ranges between 1200 and 1500 kcalories, depending on individual size and need.
T F   18.   In the exchange system of dietary control, foods listed in one group may be exchanged freely with foods listed in another group.
T F   19.   Between-meal snacks are unwise on a weight reduction diet.

Multiple Choice
        Circle the letter in front of the correct answer. Then check your answers by the test key (Appendix, p 251). Now compare all the possible answers for each item and write the following brief statements: (1) rationale for the correct answer and (2) why each one of the other responses is incorrect.

1. In human nutrition the kilocalorie is used:
   a. to measure heat energy
   b. to provide nutrients
   c. as a measure of electrical energy
   d. to control energy reactions
2. In this family of four, who has the highest energy needs per unit of body weight?
   a. the 32-year-old mother
   b. the 2-month-old son
   c. the 35-year-old father
   d. the 70-year-old grandmother
3. An overactive thyroid causes:
   a. a decreased energy need
   b. no effect on energy need
   c. increased energy need
   d. obesity because of a slower BMR
4. Which of the following foods has the highest energy value per unit of weight?
   a. potato
   b. bread
   c. meat
   d. butter
5. A slice of bread contains 2 g of protein and 15 g of carbohydrate in the form of starch. What is its caloric value?
   a. 17 kilocalories
   b. 42 kilocalories
   c. 68 kilocalories
   d. 92 kilocalories

Learning Activities

Individual Experiment: A Day's Energy Balance
Materials Scales, food value tables, food for a normal day's use.
Procedure
1. Weigh yourself and record the results
2. Convert your weight to kilograms (1 kg = 2.2 lbs)
3. Determine a day's energy requirement for your basal metabolic needs on the basis of 1 kcal/kg/hour.
4. Calculate your additional energy needs for physical activity on the basis of activities performed or general activity level [*Essentials of Nutrition and Diet Therapy*, ed 6, Table 6-1 or Clinical Application box, p 83; *Nutrition and Diet Therapy*, ed 7, Table 7-1 or Table 7-4].
5. Record your food intake for a day and calculate its total energy value, using the food tables in the appendix of your text or analyze by computer, if available, using one of the standard programs available.

Results

1.   What is your weight in pounds? In kilograms?

2.   What are your basal energy requirements? Thermic effect of food?

3.   What are your energy requirements for physical activity?

4.   What are your total energy requirements for a day? What is the total energy value of your day's food intake? Compare these two values.

5.   Are you in positive or negative energy balance? Is this reflected in your weight?

6.   Check your weight for your height in a standard height-weight table. Where do you stand?

Discussion

1.   Why is weight a reflection of energy balance?

2.   What factors would cause you to go into a negative state of energy balance and lose weight?

3.   What factors would cause you to go into a positive state of energy balance and gain weight?

Individual or Group Project: "Low-Calorie" Food Products
Materials   Note-taking materials, food products in community food market, newspaper or magazine advertisements, television commercials.
Procedure
1.   Visit an community food market and survey products that make low-calorie or weight reduction claims.
2.   List all the products found by brand name, label claims, and ingredients listed on the label.
3.   Compare in the same way the advertisements for low-calorie food products found in magazines or television commercials.

Results
1.   Evaluate each product discovered. What nutrients are modified?

2.   Compare the magazine and television advertisements as to the age group they aim at particularly. Why do you think this age is a target for such advertisements?

Discussion
1.   In light of your information and knowledge thus far, which of these advertisements do you think are truthful and sound? Would these products be helpful or useful to a person who is overweight? If so, why?

2.   Which products did you find that in your judgment are harmful or are presented by unsound advertising? Why?

3.   Do you think an overweight person should purchase food in a health food store instead of a general food market? Support your answer.

Situational Problem: Weight Control

Rosa Carlotti is a warm, outgoing 58-year-old Italian woman. She is 5 ft 2 in tall and weighs 210 lbs. Her life is centered on her large family, and she is known for her excellent Italian cooking. The family often gathers for meals, and food plays a large part in the family life.

1. Describe the state of Rosa's overall energy balance.

2. What factors do you think help to account for her situation?

3. How would the principles of energy balance help you plan a sound diet to assist her in reducing her weight?

4. What additional suggestions could you give her to increase her energy output?

5. Why would a fad diet that allows little or no carbohydrate foods and an unrestricted amount of meat proteins and fat be harmful in the long run?

Individual Food Analysis

List ten of your favorite foods. Check the caloric value of a standard portion of each item in the food value lists in the appendix of your text. Are you surprised at any of these energy values? Why?

Current Nutritional Issues

Read carefully the *Issues and Answers* article "Eating Disorders: The High Price of our Drive for Thinness" (*Essentials of Nutrition and Diet Therapy*, ed 6, p 99; *Nutrition and Diet Therapy*, ed 7, p. 167). Consider these inquiry questions:

1. Have you or someone you know ever experienced an eating disorder such as bulimia nervosa or anorexia nervosa? Can you describe the feelings and action involved?

2. What do you think some of the underlying causes are? Describe how they may lead to such abnormal attitudes and behaviors toward food and body weight.

3. Describe the compulsive overeating disorder. What is the chronic dieting syndrome? What are the dangers involved?

4. What treatment approaches are most likely to help persons with eating disorders? Describe the "stepped care" program of care.

5. What about the future? Do you see any signs of change in America's cultural attitudes or drive for unnatural thinness, especially toward women?

Chapter 7
VITAMINS

Chapter Focus

Vitamins play key roles in body metabolism and structure. They function widely to regulate cell metabolism as essential coenzyme factors, or in one special case as a hormone, and to build body structure. Since vitamins cannot be synthesized by the body, they must be supplied by the diet to avoid deficiency disease.

Summary Review Quiz

Fill in the blanks below with the appropriate number and word(s) from the list following each section. Each numbered word or phrase is used; some may be used more than once. When you have completed all the sections, check your answers for each blank by the test key (Appendix, p 251). Correct any mistakes and then review the entire chapter summary.

Fat-Soluble Vitamins

1.   A key type of function performed by many vitamins is that of _____ partner in controlling many _____ in the body. Individual vitamins have specific roles in _____. In the absence of the vitamin, a related _____ occurs, which can be cured by administration of the _____. Generally in health the vitamins are needed in very _____ amounts to perform their specific functions. Also they cannot be made by the body and are therefore dietary essentials.
2.   The vitamins soluble in _____ and not in _____ include vitamin A, D, E, and K. Vitamins are known not only by their letter names but also by their chemical names.
3.   Vitamin A's chemical name is _____ because of this association with eye disease and the _____. A deficiency of the vitamin may lead to blindness from _____, a disease affecting the _____, or to _____, a condition resulting from an inability to adjust to light and dark.

1. fat
2. retina
3. vitamin involved
4. metabolic reactions
5. cornea
6. deficiency disease
7. chemical
8. xerophthalmia
9. night blindness
10. coenzyme
11. water
12. retinol
13. body functions and structures
14. small

4.   The ultimate source of all vitamin A is a _____ called _____.
Animals and humans eat plants and convert this precursor to _____ and store it
in the _____.   Thus our diet sources of preformed vitamin A are from
_____, a small part of our total intake. The majority of our vitamin A comes
in our diet as the provitamin A in the form of _____ plant foods. The food
sources therefore include: (1) main provitamin A, the _____ in vegetables and
fruits, such as _____, squash, broccoli, _____, and apricots; and (2)
_____ vitamin A in the _____ portion of dairy products, such as butter
and cream, in liver and in egg yolk. Commercial _____ is fortified with
_____ of vitamin A per pound.
5.   Since   vitamin A is fat-soluble,, _____, _____, and
_____ are necessary for its absorption.

1. liver	6. animals	11. plant pigment
2. margarine	7. 15,000 IU	12. lipase
3. beta-carotene	8. fat	13. vitamin A
4. bile	9. preformed	14. yellow and green
5. carrots	10. sweet potatoes	

6.   Since large amounts of vitamin A can be stored, mainly in the _____,
large doses of the vitamin can be _____ and cause damage to vital tissues. This
condition of _____ causes bone and joint pains, loss of hair, and _____.
7.   Vitamin A is a component of _____, the pigment in the _____
that enables the _____ to adapt to changes in light. The chemical name of this
pigment is _____. Vitamin A also functions as a vital _____ element
necessary for the structure of healthy _____, which serves as a barrier against
_____.   Also special cells in the gums that form the _____ require
vitamin A for proper development.

1. visual purple	5. retina	9. liver
2. hypervitaminosis A	6. tooth buds	10. infection
3. eye	7. epithelial tissue	11. jaundice
4. toxic	8. growth	12. rhodopsin

8.   Vitamin D is a unique vitamin in that it occurs rarely in natural form in foods (it
is added in food processing), and the body can produce its initial compound in the
_____ on exposure to _____. Its active form as a _____ is
then produced in successive stages through the _____ and finally the _____
by special enzymes. Since this vitamin is also _____, it requires bile for
absorption. It is stored in the _____ and can also be _____ in large
amounts. This condition of _____ causes _____ of soft tissues, such as
lung and kidney, hindering their normal functions.

9.   Vitamin D's main function is associated with the minerals _____ and
_____. It is necessary for the _____ of these minerals and for their use
in _____. Thus a deficiency of vitamin D causes _____, a disease in
which the _____ do not develop properly from the softer collagenous tissue.
10.   A main carrier food for vitamin D is _____, which usually has
_____ added to each quart in processing.   Margarine is also fortified with
vitamin D.   Healthy adults get all the vitamin D they need from exposure to
_____, with the resulting synthesis of the vitamin from body _____.
Additions in the diet are needed during _____ and _____ periods.

1. liver   8. calcification   15. bone formation
2. absorption   9. phosphorus   16. calcium
3. pregnancy and lactation 10. skin   17. childhood growth
4. hypervitaminosis D   11. bones   18. cholesterol
5. 400 IU   12. sunlight   19. hormone
6. fat soluble   13. milk   20. rickets
7. kidney   14. toxic

11.   Vitamin E is the generic name of a group of vitamins, one of which,
_____, is most significant in human nutrition. It is a _____ compound
that oxidizes very slowly, giving it an important role as an _____. Its back-up
partner in this function is the trace mineral _____. Thus vitamin E protects
body lipids, especially the _____ in cell membrane structure, from
_____ and consequent deterioration. The vitamin does not have any relationship
to human _____ or _____. Its richest food sources are the
_____.   Other food sources include meat, _____, cereals, and
_____.

1. sexual potency   5. polyunsaturated fatty acids   9. reproduction
2. selenium   6. leafy vegetables   10. oxidation
3. vegetable oils   7. antioxidant   11. alpha-tocopherol
4. stable   8. eggs

12.   Vitamin K is called the _____ vitamin because of its one function of
controlling the formation of _____ in the liver. There is rarely a natural
deficiency of vitamin K, since it is synthesized by _____. This is our main
source of the vitamin. Small amounts are found in such diet items as _____ and
_____. The amount the body requires is extremely _____.

13.   Problems from a lack of vitamin K occur only in clinical situations resulting from: (1) absence of _____ to synthesize the vitamin, as in _____ and in persons having had prolonged _____ therapy; (2) lack of _____ to absorb the vitamin, and in _____ disease and surgery; (3) interference with _____ formation in the _____, as a result of _____ therapy in cardiovascular disease; and (4) impaired _____ of the vitamin in the _____ diseases affecting the _____ and its absorbing surface.

1. small
2. prothrombin
3. antibiotic
4. liver
5. intestinal

6. leafy vegetables
7. absorption
8. gallbladder
9. blood-clotting
10. mucosa

11. anticoagulant
12. intestinal bacteria
13. bile
14. newborn infants

Discussion Questions

1.   Explain what is meant by coenzyme function. Give an example.

2.   What is an antimetabolite? How does the drug bishydroxycoumarin (Dicumarol) act in this way? What is its effect as a result?

3.   Why would a person lacking vitamin A be more prone to develop recurrent urinary tract or eye infections?

4.   How would you advise a person taking megadoses of vitamin A?

5.   A tendency toward internal bleeding occurs in advanced liver disease such as cirrhosis. Would vitamin K therapy be effective in such cases? Explain your answer.

6.   Why would a person on a high polyunsaturated fat diet for heart disease require more vitamin E?

Self-Test Questions

<u>True-False</u>
Circle the "T" if a statement is true and write a brief rationale for its accuracy. If it is false, circle the "F" and write the correct statement.

T F 1.   A coenzyme acts alone to control a specific metabolic reaction.
T F 2.   Carotene is preformed vitamin A found in animal food sources.
T F 3.   Vitamin A is water soluble and hence is found in the nonfat part of milk.
T F 4.   Visual purple is a pigment in the retina of the eye associated with color blindness.
T F 5.   Vitamin D and sufficient dietary calcium and phosphorus prevent rickets.
T F 6.   With exposure to sunlight, vitamin D hormone can be made from cholesterol in the skin and a special activating enzyme in the kidney.
T F 7.   There is no danger in toxic amounts of any of the fat-soluble vitamins.
T F 8.   Vitamin K is found in meat, especially liver, as well as in green leafy vegetables.

<u>Multiple Choice</u>
Circle the letter in front of the correct answer. Then check your answers by the test key (Appendix, p 252). Now compare all the possible answers for each item and write the following brief statements: (1) rationale for the correct answer and (2) why each one of the other responses is incorrect.

1.   Vitamin A is a fat-soluble vitamin produced by humans and other animals from its precursor, carotene, or provitamin A—a green and yellow plant pigment—and then stored in the body. Hence our main sources of this vitamin include:
    (1)   nonfat milk
    (2)   leafy green vegetables
    (3)   carrots
    (4)   oranges
    (5)   butter
    (6)   tomatoes
    a.   1, 2, and 4
    b.   2, 3, and 5
    c.   1, 3, and 6
    d.   3, 4, and 5
2.   Because vitamin A is fat-soluble, it requires a helping agent for absorption. This agent is:
    a.   lipase
    b.   amylase
    c.   hydrochloric acid
    d.   bile

3.	Megadoses of vitamin A being advocated by some persons must be questioned because:
	a.	it cannot be stored, and the excess amount would saturate the general body tissues
	b.	it is highly toxic even in small amounts
	c.	the liver has a great storage capacity for the vitamin, even to toxic amounts
	d.	although the body's requirement for the vitamin is large, the cells can synthesize more as needed

4.	The vision cycle in the eye requires vitamin A. Here the vitamin functions as:
	a.	a necessary component of visual purple, which controls light and dark adaptation
	b.	a part of the retina that controls color blindness
	c.	the material in the cornea that prevents cataract formation
	d.	an integral part of the retina's black pigment, melanin, which prevents excessive light reflection

5.	Vitamin D is formed from a cholesterol base that is converted to a final active hormone in the:
	a.	liver
	b.	skin
	c.	kidney
	d.	intestinal wall

6.	The structure of vitamin E provides an active site for taking up oxygen; hence it acts as an antioxidant to other vulnerable substances, especially certain lipids and fat-related compounds. This antioxidant property has given vitamin E an essential role in human nutrition as a:
	a.	a support therapy in cardiovascular disease
	b.	protector of lipid cell membrane structures
	c.	necessary agent for sexual potency and reproductive process
	d.	surface medication to prevent skin odors and wound scars

7.	Which of the following statements are true about the sources of vitamin K?
	a.	Vitamin K is found in a wide variety of foods so there is no danger of a deficiency.
	b.	Vitamin K can easily be absorbed without assistance so we are assured of getting into our systems all that we consume.
	c.	Vitamin K is rarely found in dietary food sources so a natural deficiency can easily occur.
	d.	Most of our vitamin K required for metabolic needs is produced by intestinal bacteria.

Learning Activities

Individual or Group Project: Regular and Megadose Use of Vitamin Pills
Procedure
1.   Interview a small sample of persons to determine:
        a.   How many are purchasing and using low-dosage pills of any vitamins and,
                if so, what vitamins they are using, in what amounts, and their reasons for
                using them.
        b.   How many are using regular strength vitamin pills, and, if so, which ones
                and their reasons for taking them.
2.   Interview several clerks in drugstores concerning any increase in sales of such
        vitamin pills and, if so, why they think that this is happening.
3.   Visit a health food store, posing as a potential customer. Inquire about vitamin
        pills, different potencies, and possible benefits. Look carefully at the stock,
        reading labels and advertisements. Ask for any literature (booklets, pamphlets,
        advertisements sheets) to take with you to study and give to friends.
4.   Survey vitamin advertisements in magazines, in newspapers, or on television.

Results
1.   List the responses to your interview survey questions. Total like responses from
        each of your project group members.

2.   Describe your encounter at the health food stores.

3.   What claims did you find in the magazines and television advertisements?

Discussion
1.   Evaluate the results of your survey on the use of vitamin pills.

2.   Evaluate the claims that you discovered at the health food store.

3.   What claims did you find in the magazines and television advertisements?

Discussion
1.   Evaluate the results of your survey on the use of vitamin pills.

2.   Evaluate the claims that you discovered at the health food store.

3.   What was the "pitch" of the magazine and television advertisements?

4.   What valid use do you think vitamin supplements have?

Situational Problem
       The following three patients are located in separate clinical areas of the hospital.
Surgical ward   Mrs. Jones has just returned from surgery after having had a cholecystectomy for gallstones. Her dressing over the surgical incision requires close watching and possibly frequent changes.
Medical ward   Mr. Roberts is gradually recovering from a heart attach caused by the fatty plaques in the coronary vessels supplying blood to his heart muscle and the formation of a blood clot that cut off the blood supply to part of the tissue. As part of his therapy his physician has placed him on bishydroxycoumarin for anticoagulant therapy. His blood-clotting time will be closely monitored and an antidote kept at hand for use as needed.
Nursery   Baby girl Smith is only a few hours old. Part of her immediate routine care after birth included administration of an important control agent to prevent hemorrhage.
1.   What common control agent is involved in each of these cases? What is its basic action?

2.   Describe the source of the problem with this control agent in each case. Although this common agent is involved, the cause of the problem with this substance is different in each case.

3.   What antidote would be kept available if needed for Mr. Roberts?

<u>Night blindness</u>   Mr. Jackson is worried about losing his job as a truck driver because he is having increasing difficulty in seeing the road and road signs at night. When he visits his physician and has his vision tested, he learns that he has developed night blindness.

1.   What is the control agent involved? How is this agent involved in Mr. Jackson's vision problem?

2.   What foods would you suggest that Mr. Jackson increase in his diet? What form of the agent does each of the foods contain?

Individual Diet Analysis: Vitamin A

Record in detail your food intake for a day, including all meal and snack items. Use the Daily Food Intake box on p 294 to list your day's food and check each item containing vitamin A. Calculate your total vitamin A intake for the day. Compare your intake with the Recommended Dietary Allowance (RDA) for vitamin A.

1.   How does your intake compare with the RDA standard?

2.   What foods could you add to increase your intake?

Summary Review Quiz

Fill in the blanks below with the appropriate number and word(s) from the list following each section. Each numbered word or phrase is used: some may be used more than once. When you have completed all the sections, check your answers for each blank by the test key (Appendix, p 253). Correct any mistakes and then review the entire chapter summary.

Water-Soluble Vitamins

1.   Vitamin C is soluble in _____ but not in _____. It is a chemically _____ and an easily _____ acid. Its chemical name is _____ because of its properties in curing _____. Because of its chemical properties, vitamin C is easily lost if care is not taken in _____ and _____ of food sources.

2.   Since it is _____ soluble, vitamin C is easily _____ in the small intestine. It is not stored in the body and must be obtained in the _____.

1. scurvy	5. unstable	9. daily diet
2. oxidized	6. fat	10. ascorbic acid
3. absorbed	7. storing	
4. cooking	8. water	

3.   Vitamin C's main function is to deposit a _____ between cells. Hence it is a necessary agent to _____, especially for the development of ground substance into _____. For example, without vitamin C _____ weaken and rupture easily, causing easy bruising, general tissue _____, poor _____, and soft _____ with loosened teeth. A major effect of vitamin C deficiency disease, _____, is diffuse, widespread, internal _____. Vitamin C also helps hemoglobin formation by aiding the absorption of _____.

4.   Extra vitamin C is needed for _____ and normal tissue _____ of any kind. It also helps body tissue resist _____. Adequate amounts for these needs do not require megadoses of vitamin C advocated by some persons. The excess beyond _____ and daily need cannot be stored and is excreted in the _____.

5.   The main food source of vitamin C is _____. Good additional sources are found in a variety of vegetables and fruits, including _____, _____, green and chili peppers, leafy vegetables, and broccoli.

1. scurvy	7. wound healing	13. cementing substance
2. blood capillary membranes	8. potatoes	14. urine
3. iron	9. growth	15. tissue hemorrhage
4. tissue saturation	10. tomatoes	16. collagen
5. build tissue	11. infection	17. bleeding gums
6. citrus fruit	12. bleeding	

6.   Thiamin is a key control agent in the metabolism of _____. It is a necessary _____ in ky reactions that produce _____ from _____ or convert _____ to _____ for tissue use and storage. Its deficiency causes the disease _____, which is characterized by _____, gastrointestinal and _____ disturbances, and _____. If the process continues, _____ may result.

7.   The requirement for thiamin increases as the _____ requirement in terms of _____ increases. Such increases would be needed in periods of _____, _____, larger body size, _____, and chronic illness. Food sources of thiamin include _____, especially _____, whole or enriched _____, and legumes. A deficiency of thiamin is quite possible because it is _____ in food than some of the other vitamins.

1. glucose	7. pork	13. grains
2. paralysis	8. muscle weakness	14. fevers and infections
3. pregnancy	9. less widely distributed	15. energy
4. fat	10. lean meat	16. nerve irritability
5. kilocalories	11. cardiovascular	17. growth
6. coenzyme	12. carbohydrate	18. beriberi

8.   Riboflavin is so named because it contains the sugar _____ and its main yellow pigment found in _____. It functions as an important coenzyme in _____ metabolism for energy production and in _____ metabolism for tissue building. Thus riboflavin deficiency is often manifested in _____ and breakdown. The requirement for riboflavin is related to _____, metabolic activity, and _____, all of which involve _____ metabolism, and to increased _____ that requires more _____ metabolism. Its main food sources are _____ and _____. Cereals are a source only if they are _____.

1. carbohydrate	5. milk whey	9. milk
2. rate of growth	6. energy	10. ribose
3. enriched	7. body size	11. exercise
4. tissue inflammation	8. organ meats	12. protein

9.   Niacin was discovered in the search for the cure for _____. It is the specific _____ factor whose absence in the diet causes the disease. It is related to the _____ amino acid _____, which is precursor of the vitamin. Thus the requirement of the vitamin is stated in terms of _____ to cover food sources of both the _____ and of _____.

10.   Niacin is a partner with _____ in a key _____ role in cell energy systems. Deficiency symptoms include general _____, a specific _____ in which the skin becomes darkened and scaly, and _____ problems such as neuritis, confusion, and disorientation. A major food source of niacin is _____. Other sources include peanuts, legumes, and _____.

1. niacin equivalents
2. central nervous system
3. essential
4. riboflavin

5. meat
6. pellagra
7. weakness
8. preformed vitamin

9. enriched cereals
10. coenzyme
11. dermatitis
12. tryptophan

11.   Pyridoxine is an active _____ factor in many reactions governing the use of _____ in the body. These reactions move _____ from one compound to another to form new _____ or release _____. In this role it helps to produce the non-protein _____, which is an essential part of _____. Pyridoxine also aids _____ by serving as a _____. Food sources of the vitamin include _____, corn, and meats, especially _____.

12.   Pantothenic acid is _____ in all living things and is synthesized in considerable amount by _____, so its deficiency is unlikely. It is an _____ of a key activating enzyme in a large number of metabolic reactions, especially in _____.

1. carrier
2. widespread
3. amino acids
4. energy production
5. hemoglobin

6. energy
7. wheat
8. amino acid absorption
9. coenzyme
10. intestinal bacteria

11. liver
12. heme
13. essential component
14. nitrogen

13.   Folic acid is an important _____ factor, discovered in the study of _____. It serves an essential _____ function in the production of cell nucleus material and of the _____ portion of _____. A deficiency of folic acid produces a specific _____ in which _____ red blood cells are formed. These cells cannot carry _____ properly. Increased amounts of folic acid are required in _____, since fetal development increases the demand for the vitamin. Folic acid is also an effective treatment in the intestinal disease _____. Food sources include _____ and _____.

1. large immature
2. oxygen
3. anemias
4. hemoglobin

5. leafy vegetables
6. coenzyme
7. megaloblastic anemia
8. sprue

9. liver
10. blood-forming
11. pregnancy
12. heme

14. Vitamin B_{12} is named_____ because of its unique structure with _____ at the center. It is the specific control agent to prevent _____. Food sources of the vitamin are all of _____ origin—_____, especially liver, milk, egg, and cheese—since it is synthesized in the animal's gastrointestinal tract by microorganisms. Hence only _____ are likely to experience a real deficiency state of the vitamin.

15. Vitamin B_{12} requires two _____ for absorption. It is prepared in a free form by _____ and combined for absorption with _____, a mucoprotein substance in the gastric juices, as a _____. The defect, therefore, in pernicious anemia is at the point of B_{12} _____ because of the lack of this _____. Therefore pernicious anemia must be treated by _____ of B_{12} to bypass the _____ defect. Vitamin B_{12} functions as a _____ in the formation of hemoglobin, probably indirectly by activating _____. Pernicious anemia may develop in situations such as (1) _____ when there is a general reduction of gastric secretions and hence of their component _____ or (2) in clinical problems after _____ (surgical removal of the stomach), which would eliminate the _____. Because of this broad role in body metabolism, vitamin B_{12} is _____ in active body tissue, especially the _____.

1. gastric secretions
2. animal
3. injections
4. folic acid
5. cobalt
6. gastrectomy
7. liver
8. true vegetarians
9. intrinsic factor
10. coenzyme
11. cobalamin
12. carrier
13. stored widely
14. absorption
15. hydrochloric acid
16. lean meat
17. aging
18. pernicious anemia

Discussion Questions

1. Why would increased amount of vitamin C be needed after a severe body injury such as might be sustained in a car accident?

2. Capillary walls are thin, single-cell membranes. Tissue bleeding is the primary symptom of vitamin C deficiency. How are these two statements related?

3. Account for the symptom of thiamin deficiency related to the function of the gastrointestinal tract and the central nervous system.

4.	If pellagra is caused by niacin deficiency, why does milk, which is low in niacin, cure it? What is a *niacin equivalent*?

5.	What is the relationship of folic acid and B_{12} to anemia?

Self-Test Questions

True-False
Circle the "T" if a statement is true and write a brief rationale for its accuracy. If it is false, circle the "F" and write the correct statement.

T F 1. Connective tissue such as collagen requires vitamin C for its formation.

T F 2. Extra vitamin C is stored in the liver to meet the demands of tissue infections.

T F 3. Freshly squeezed orange juice may be kept indefinitely in the refrigerator without any loss of vitamin C.

T F 4. The dietary requirements for thiamin are stated in relation to energy needs, as expressed in caloric intake.

T F 5. A deficiency of thiamin is unlikely, since it is widespread in a variety of food sources.

T F 6. The main food source of riboflavin is milk.

T F 7. The deficiency disease associated with the discovery of niacin is beriberi.

T F 8. Vitamin B_6 (pyridoxine) is required as a carrier to aid the absorption of fatty acids.

T F 9. Pantothenic acid is a vital component of active acetyl-coenzyme A, the important common molecule in the process of energy production in the cell.

T F 10. A deficiency of vitamin B_{12} is rare because it is found in a number of plant and animal food sources.

Multiple Choice
Circle the letter in front of the correct answer. Then check your answers by the test key (Appendix, p 254). Now compare all the possible answers for each item and write the following brief statements: (1) rationale for the correct answer and (2) why each one of the other responses is incorrect.

1.	Vitamin C has been advocated in megadoses to prevent infections such as the common cold. Which of the following chemical characteristics of the vitamin would seem to refute these claims?

    a.	Vitamin C is a complex compound of high molecular weight and hence unavailable metabolically in such large amounts.

b.   Storage organs of the body such as the liver or adipose tissue can accumulate large storage reserves of the vitamin.

c.   When general tissue saturation levels are reached, the rest of the vitamin is excreted in the urine.

d.   Vitamin C is fat-soluble, and hence excess becomes bound in fat compounds and is unavailable in the body.

2. Vitamin C in human nutrition is related to tissue integrity and hemorrhagic disease. It controls both because it:

    a.   preserves the structural integrity of tissue by protecting the lipid matrix of cell membranes from oxidation

    b.   prevents tissue hemorrhage by providing essential blood-clotting materials

    c.   facilitates adequate absorption of calcium and phosphorus for bone formation to prevent bleeding in the joints

    d.   strengthens capillary membranes and structural tissue through depositing cementing material to build collagen from ground substance

3. If you found on diet analysis of a clinic patient that he was lacking in vitamin C, which of the following foods would you suggest he add to increase in his diet?

    a.   fortified margarine

    b.   enriched cereals, grains, and breads

    c.   fortified milk

    d.   fresh green vegetables and citrus fruit

4. Thiamin plays a key metabolic role as cell coenzyme factor in glucose oxidation. This vital role links thiamin to carbohydrate and fat metabolism and energy production. Hence deficiencies of thiamin may be manifested by:

    a.   increased gastrointestinal secretion and muscle action

    b.   weakened heart muscle, sometimes leading to cardiac failure

    c.   contraction of smooth muscle of blood vessels, causing edema of the extremities

    d.   nerve irritation caused by excess fat covering of nerve fibers

5. Thiamin is an important part of nutritional therapy for patients with alcoholism because the malnutrition associated with alcohol abuse leads to:

    a.   vision problems

    b.   bone disease

    c.   neurologic problems

    d.   hemorrhagic disorders

6. Two materials in gastric secretions are necessary for the absorption of vitamin B_{12}. When one or both are absent, pernicious anemia results. These materials are:

    a.   hydrochloric acid and intrinsic factor

    b.   pepsin and gastric lipase

    c.   iron and folic acid

    d.   ascorbic acid and pantothenic acid

Learning Activities

<u>Situational Problems</u>

<u>Pregnancy</u> Betty, a young teen-ager, is pregnant with her first child. Because of her age, she has been referred to the high-risk prenatal clinic. You are discussing with her the importance of her diet.

1. Name four particular vitamins (two fat soluble and two water soluble) that you would especially stress as necessary in good amounts during her pregnancy. What reasons could you give her for this need in each case?

2. For each of these vitamins, what sources would you suggest to Betty that she use in increased amounts?

<u>Burns</u> A patient with extensive severe burns is carefully watched in the first few days of the shock and recovery phases. Now that he is beginning to eat, the clinical nutritionist outlines a diet high in kilocalories, protein, and vitamins. Although the patient's appetite is poor, successful nutritional therapy is vital to his recovery.

1. What two vitamins would merit special attention in this case? Give your reasons in each case.

2. What are the reasons for the accompanying increased need for protein and kilocalories?

3. What foods would our use to supply additional amounts of these vitamins?

<u>Surgery</u> After several years of intractable peptic ulcer disease, Mr. Brown has had a total gastrectomy. Sometime later he develops a severe anemia.

1. What type of anemia does Mr. Brown probably have? What vitamin is involved basically in this problem?

2. What caused Mr. Brown's anemia to develop?

3. What treatment would be given? Why?

Alcoholism A malnourished man has been brought into the emergency room suffering from mental confusion and psychosis—delirium tremens. His malnutrition from excessive alcohol intake has brought about degenerative changes in the peripheral nerves and the nerve cells of the cerebral cortex. When he is able to eat, he is given large amounts of carbohydrates and vitamins.
1. What particular vitamin does this man need in large amounts? Why?

2. What relation does this vitamin have to the increased intake of carbohydrate?

Neurologic disability A malnourished Chinese refugee boy has been living mainly on polished rice. He is brought into the hospital with tingling and numbness in his extremities and increasing inability to use his legs.
1. What control agent is lacking in his diet and mainly responsible for his neuromuscular symptoms? What is this disease?

2. What is the action of this control agent and how does this relate to his symptoms?

3. Besides large therapeutic doses of the vitamin involved, what foods would you try to increase in his diet to support his recovery?

Dermatitis Before grain enrichment became widespread, poor persons in the rural South who subsisted mainly on corn and cornmeal developed a disease characterized by a particular kind of skin eruption—a dark, scaly dermatitis, especially sensitive to sunlight. As the disease progressed, they developed neuritis and became increasingly apathetic and disoriented.

1. What is the disease and its cause? What is the action of the control agent involved? How does this related to the symptoms of the disease?

2. Why would diets almost exclusively of corn cause this disease?

3. What foods should be increased in the diet to prevent this disease?

Current Nutritional Issues

Read carefully the *Issues and Answers* article "Guidelines for Vitamin Supplementation" (*Essentials of Nutrition and Diet Therapy*, ed 6, p 132; *Clinical applications* box, *Nutrition and Diet Therapy*, ed 7, p 215). Consider these inquiry questions:

1. What factors do you think support the large vitamin supplementation industry and practices? How do these feed on each other?

2. In what situations, if any, of your own or others' experiences have you found such supplementation valid? Describe and support your response.

3. What does the term "biochemical individuality" mean? Why does this make individual assessment an important practice?

4. Review carefully the conditions listed here in relation to the question of vitamin supplementation. In light of your present knowledge, what is your own view of need in each case and how would you advise a client or patient? Research each situation further in your text or journals to expand your review.

Chapter 8
MINERALS

Chapter Focus

The widely distributed natural inorganic minerals have equally broad and varied key roles in body metabolism as coenzyme factors and structural material. The requirements of these essential nutrient components also vary widely from relatively large amounts of major minerals to minute quantities of trace elements.

Summary-Review Quiz

Fill in the blanks below with the appropriate number and word(s) from the list following each section. Each numbered word or phrase is used; some may be used more than once. When you have completed all the sections, check your answers for each blank by the test key (Appendix, p 254). Correct any mistakes and then review the entire chapter summary.

<u>Major Minerals</u>
1. Although the body's minerals are single _____ rather than complex _____ like the vitamins, they help to regulate and control a wide variety of _____. They are usually classified according to the _____ of each mineral needed to perform its functions.
2. Seven _____ minerals are clearly _____ to human life and function: _____, magnesium, _____, sulfur, _____, _____, and chlorine. Ten _____ minerals are definitely _____ elements: _____, copper, _____, manganese, cobalt, _____, selenium, _____, fluoride, and molybdenum. Eight additional _____ minerals are probably _____ elements, though their status still awaits better means of _____, because body tissue amounts are so _____. These elements are _____, boron, _____, cadmium, nickel, _____, vanadium, and arsenic.

1. amount
2. zinc
3. calcium
4. trace
5. organic compounds
6. small
7. sodium
8. tin
9. essential
10. analysis
11. silicon
12. phosphorus
13. inorganic elements
14. iodine
15. aluminum
16. body functions
17. iron
18. major
19. chromium
20. potassium

3.   The mineral present in the body in the largest amount is _____. Almost all of it is in the _____, but the small remaining 1% in the _____ is vital. The body's overall intake-output _____ is controlled mainly at the point of _____ by _____ and other factors such as body need. Only a _____ amount of the total _____ taken in is absorbed.

4.   In health, the amount of this major mineral in the bone tissue is in constant _____ with the small amount of it in the _____. In certain bone diseases, such as _____, or when the body is _____, as in a body cast, an excess of this major mineral is withdrawn from the _____.

1. absorption	5. osteoporosis	9. calcium
2. small	6. calcium balance	10. immobile
3. dynamic turnover balance	7. bones	11. blood
4. bone tissue	8. vitamin D hormone	12. dietary calcium

5.   The _____ amount of free ionized _____ calcium has several important functions. It aids _____, transmission of nerve impulses, _____, _____ permeability, and activation of _____.

6.   The amount of serum calcium is always maintained in a constant relationship with _____. This is called the _____. When the serum level of _____ increases, therefore, the calcium level _____. This causes symptoms of _____ —muscle jerking and spasms—because calcium is necessary for normal _____. To help prevent such imbalance, the serum calcium level is governed by a special control agent, the _____. Thus two agents work as partners to regulate the _____: (1) _____, which mainly governs absorption and bone deposit, and (2) _____, which mainly governs bone withdrawal and urinary phosphorus excretion.

1. enzymes	5. blood	9. small
2. decreases	6. phosphorus	10. membrane
3. muscle action	7. tetany	11. serum calcium-phosphorus balance
4. vitamin D hormone	8. parathyroid hormone	12. blood clotting

7.   Calcium's partner in _____ is phosphorus. Its balance in the body is controlled by the same agents, _____ and _____. It combines with calcium to form _____. It is found in many of the same _____ sources. However, it differs from calcium in its major overall _____ function. In cell metabolism, phosphorus is vital in _____, and in the blood it maintains a _____ system to help control _____ balance. As a result of these general tissue functions, another food source of phosphorus is _____.

1. food
2. vitamin D hormone
3. lean meat
4. parathyroid hormone
5. energy production
6. metabolic
7. bone metabolism
8. acid-base
9. buffer
10. bones and teeth

8.   The major amount of body sodium is in _____ form. Because minerals in this _____ state can carry an _____, the are called _____. Sodium carries a _____ charge and is called a _____. Its major function is to guard _____ balance _____ the cells. It also provides the _____ in the body's major _____ system. In addition, sodium ions help to move substances across cell membranes and to maintain normal _____.

9.   Since the main route of sodium excretion is the _____, the major sodium-guarding agent operates there in the _____ to control the amount of sodium _____ or excreted. This control agent is _____, a major hormone produced by the _____ upon stimulation by _____ action.

10.   Dietary sodium intake varies widely according to the amount of _____ used in food. Sources of sodium include _____, meat, eggs, and a few _____. No appreciable amount of natural sodium occurs in _____.

1. positive
2. base partner
3. reabsorbed
4. muscle action
5. water
6. vegetables
7. electrical charge
8. renin-angiotensin
9. kidney
10. fruit
11. cation
12. milk
13. nephrons
14. free ionized
15. aldosterone
16. outside
17. electrolytes
18. salt
19. adrenal glands
20. acid-base buffer

11.   The major amount of body potassium also exists in the _____ form. It serves as the major _____ inside the _____ to balance with sodium outside the _____ in maintaining the body's _____. The _____ also controls blood potassium by means of the _____ mechanism. Under this hormonal control, sodium is reabsorbed by the _____ and potassium is _____ in exchange to maintain the balance between the two electrolytes.

12.   In balance with sodium, potassium not only helps to guard _____ but also regulates _____, especially that of the _____. As a result, changes in serum potassium level are reflected immediately in changes in the rate of the _____. Uncontrolled potassium loss in body fluids as in prolonged _____ and dehydration could lead to serious complications of _____.

13.   Potassium is needed also for the storage of _____ in the liver and of _____ in muscle _____ and cell _____. Potassium is _____ distributed in foods so that diet usually contains _____ for normal needs.

1. heart beat	7. muscle action	13. nitrogen
2. kidney	8. nephrons	14. aldosterone
3. ample amount	9. cation	15. protein
4. excreted	10. widely	16. water balance
5. cardiac arrest	11. diarrhea	17. glycogen
6. cells	12. free ionized	18. heart muscle

Trace Elements

1.   Of the trace minerals, iron is most significant as a _____ factor. It is the core component of _____, the _____ part of _____, the component in _____ that carries _____ to the tissue for cell oxidation and metabolism.

2.   Dietary iron occurs in two forms: _____ and _____. The larger portion by far is the _____ portion that comes from _____ of the plant sources and _____ of the animal sources. Of the two forms of dietary iron, the larger _____ portion is absorbed much more slowly because it is tightly bound in _____. This fact is of nutritional concern because we eat far more _____ iron foods than _____ iron ones.

1. nonprotein	5. red blood cells	9. nonheme
2. oxygen	6. organic compounds	10. hemoglobin
3. heme	7. 100%	
4. 60%	8. blood-building	

3.   Iron cannot be _____ in its natural food form so it must be prepared for _____ by gastric _____. The amount of dietary iron _____ is controlled by a protein-iron compound in the intestinal mucosa called _____. Only a small amount of the _____ is actually absorbed, the amount depending mainly on _____, as in _____ states or growth and _____ demands. The amount absorbed also depends on the presence of _____ to prepare it and binding agents or hindering substances. Iron absorption is also aided by _____.

4.   After absorption the body carefully maintains and conserves its overall blood-tissues-hemoglobin _____. As the cell _____ is broken down, the iron is _____ for use over and over again.

1. pregnancy
2. absorption
3. recycled
4. body need

5. ferritin
6. Vitamin C
7. hemoglobin
8. hydrochloric acid

9. deficiency
10. iron balance
11. absorbed
12. dietary iron

5.   A deficiency of iron leads to _____. The cause of the deficiency determines the type of _____. It may be caused by _____ iron deficiency in the _____, by _____, by lack of _____, or by _____ diseases.

6.   Older infants or _____ fed only _____ and insufficient additional _____ may develop a typical _____ because _____ does not contain iron and _____ are depleted. Iron _____ during the life cycle are greatest for _____ during the _____, especially during _____.

1. loss of blood
2. solid foods
3. anemia
4. toddlers
5. milk anemia

6. malabsorption
7. diet
8. fetal stores
9. pregnancy
10. gastric hydrochloric acid

11. women
12. nutritional anemia
13. reproductive years
14. milk
15. requirements
16. primary

7.   Iodine is a _____ mineral with one function. It provides the _____ with major component for producing its hormone _____. The amount of _____ iodine taken up by the _____ is controlled by the hormone _____ from the body's master gland, the _____. After the iodine-containing hormone _____ is produced by the _____, the hormone is released to the _____ and carried to the tissues to regulate _____. Iodine is needed especially in _____ periods such as _____ and _____, when _____ are increased because of increased cell work.

1. blood
2. plasma
3. BMR
4. pituitary

5. pregnancy
6. thyroid gland
7. metabolic needs
8. thyroxine

9. rapid growth
10. adolescence
11. trace
12. TSH

8.   The classic disease resulting from _____ of iodine is _____. The _____ enlarges because it overworks, trying to obtain sufficient iodine from the _____ supply in the _____.

9.   Natural plant food sources of iodine vary widely, depending on the _____ of the mineral. Some iodine is contributed by _____. The main dietary source, however, is _____. Thus this commercial _____ program is important. Consumers should check _____ on _____ to be sure the product has been _____.

1. soil content
2. decreased
3. enrichment
4. goiter

5. labels
6. iodized salt
7. seafood
8. thyroid gland

9. iodized
10. dietary deficiency
11. salt
12. blood

10.   Zinc is a trace element with widespread _____ functions as a _____ factor, especially in _____. Persons particularly at risk for a _____ of zinc are _____ patients with chronic illnesses and _____. They have _____, poor appetites, and _____ from their illness and the added problems of _____ defects, which contribute to nutritional deficiency.

11.   Fluoride is a trace mineral associated with _____. Fluoride treatment of developing teeth during childhood largely prevents _____. Consequently public health authorities recommend community _____ as a preventive measure.

1. surgery
2. deficiency
3. taste and smell
4. dental health

5. coenzyme
6. elderly
7. dental caries
8. unhealed wounds

9. metabolic
10. limited diets
11. water fluoridation
12. tissue healing

Water-Electrolyte Balance
1.   Overall body water balance is maintained by three interdependent factors:
(1) the _____, (2) the various _____, and (3) the _____ throughout the body that control their flow.
2.   The adult body is about _____ water. Water is essential to life. It provides the necessary _____ for _____, it gives _____ to the body, and it provides the means for maintaining _____.
3.   Total body water exists in two main divisions or collective _____, according to its distribution inside or outside the cells. The total water outside the cells is called _____, and the total water inside the cells is called _____. The amount of water _____ is about _____ the amount of water _____.

1. 65%
2. compartments
3. cell metabolism
4. intercellular fluid (ICF)
5. particles in solution

6. outside cells
7. form and structure
8. twice
9. total body water
10. extracellular fluid (ECF)

11. inside cells
12. separating membranes
13. body temperature
14. internal environment

4.   Water comes into the body system in three ways: _____, _____, and water produced by _____. Water leaves the body through the _____, the _____, the _____, and a small amount in the _____. This water _____ must be a constant _____ to prevent _____.

5.   The particles in solution in body water control its _____. These particulates are called _____. The two main types are _____ and _____.

1. plasma protein
2. dehydration
3. intake and output
4. water in food
5. lungs
6. electrolytes
7. kidneys
8. balance
9. skin
10. solutes
11. water in beverages
12. distribution
13. cell metabolism
14. feces

6.   Several body minerals provide the major _____ for the body. These particles are small _____ that move easily in solution and carry either _____, in which case they are called cations, or _____, in which case they are called anions. The main cation guarding the water outside the cell is _____. The main cation guarding the water inside the cell is _____. Because _____ are small, they can _____ across most body membranes and hence control _____.

7.   Plasma protein, mainly in the form of _____, is an organic compound _____ in size than the electrolytes. Because of its size, these molecules _____ freely across capillary membranes and are retained in the _____. Thus the plasma protein protects blood _____ by maintaining sufficient _____ to pull tissue water constantly back into _____. This basic _____ mechanism governed by the _____ from plasma protein is called the _____ mechanism. It is the body's major means of maintaining _____ and normal _____.

1. diffuse freely
2. albumin
3. sodium
4. volume
5. capillary circulation
6. ions
7. do not diffuse
8. tissue fluid circulation
9. negative electrical charges
10. larger
11. water balance
12. electrolytes
13. colloidal osmotic pressure
14. potassium
15. positive electrical charges
16. blood vessels
17. capillary fluid shift
18. water movement

8.   The two types of separating membranes that control water and solute flow are the _____ membrane and the _____ membrane. The _____ membrane is thin and porous so water and its solutes, except for _____, move freely across it according to respective _____ differences. The _____ membrane is a thicker construction of fat and protein designed to protect the cell and its contents. Special receptors and _____ are necessary to carry materials across it.

9. Forces that help move water and solutes across membranes include _____, _____, _____, _____, and _____.

1. plasma protein
2. diffusion
3. transport mechanisms
4. filtration

5. capillary
6. osmosis
7. concentration
8. active transport

9. pinocytosis
10. cell

10. Two hormonal controls help maintain water balance. These are _____, a hormone from the _____ gland, which conserves _____ by increasing its _____ by the _____, and _____, a hormone from the _____ glands, which conserves _____ by increasing its _____.

11. In addition to normal balance activities, both these hormonal mechanisms are _____ by body stress situations such as injury or _____. Normally these hormonal mechanisms are life-saving _____ controls. However, they are also triggered in clinical disease problems such as _____. In this case, they only serve to make matters worse because the failing _____ cannot maintain the normal amount of _____ output.

1. water
2. aldosterone
3. reabsorption
4. pituitary
5. congestive heart failure

6. kidneys
7. blood
8. increased
9. ADH
10. heart muscle

11. surgery
12. sodium
13. homeostatic
14. adrenal

Discussion Questions

1. Why is phosphorus called the *metabolic twin* of calcium? In what functions does this description apply? In what functions does it not apply?

2. What are the two control agents that govern calcium and phosphorus balance in the body? How do they operate together? Would this be an example of biologic synergism? Why? On what basis should you reclassify vitamin D as a hormone?

3. Why would a person wearing a large body cast for a broken back need to drink more water daily and not drink excessive amounts of milk?

4. What is the significance of the capillary fluid shift mechanism in overall body water balance? Give several examples of its operation. What do you think would happen to the serum potassium level after massive burns? Why would potassium replacement *not* be given immediately, but only later as needed?

5. Why would nutritional anemia probably develop after a total gastrectomy?

6. What is the "iron cost" of pregnancy? Why is iron significant at this time?

7. Hemoglobin synthesis requires a number of specific nutrients. Name as many of these nutrients as you can and describe what each one does.

8. What is meant by the term *negative feedback mechanism*? How does this action apply in thyroxine synthesis?

Self-Test Questions

True-False

Circle the "T" if a statement is true and write a brief rationale for its accuracy. If it is false, circle the "F" and write the correct statement.

T F 1. Calcium must be prepared for absorption by hydrochloric acid in the gastric secretion.

T F 2. The majority of calcium in the diet is absorbed and used by the body for bone formation.

T F 3. Bone calcium and serum calcium are maintained in a constant interdependent balance.

T F 4. The average adult use of sodium is about 10 times the amount the body actually requires for metabolic balance.

T F 5. Edema is a condition in which fluid is decreased in the tissues.

T F 6. Chloride is the major anion in body water outside the cells

T F 7. Sulfur contributes important structural bonds to certain proteins.

T F 8. Most of the dietary iron is absorbed, and the body's iron balance is then controlled by urinary excretion.

T F 9. Liver is the body's main iron storage site.

T F 10. Iron is widespread in food sources so a deficiency problem is rare.

T F 11. Vitamin C aids iron absorption.

T F 12. Iron is constantly lost with short-lived red cells and must therefore be replaced from newly absorbed dietary iron and liver storage.

T F 13. Hemorrhagic anemia is caused by a dietary deficiency of iron.

T F 14. The best food source of iron is milk.

T F 15. Iodine has many metabolic functions, the most important of which is its role in thyroxine synthesis.

T F 16. Thyroxine is synthesized by the pituitary gland.

T F 17. Dental caries can be largely prevented by the use of small amounts of fluorine.

Multiple Choice

Circle the letter in front of the correct answer. Then check your answers by the test key (Appendix, p 256). Now compare all the possible answers for each item and write the following brief statements: (1) rationale for the correct answer and (2) why each one of the other responses is wrong.

1. Overall calcium balance in the body is maintained by two sets of balances: (1) absorption-excretion, regulating the amount that will be absorbed, and (2) depositing-mobilizing as bone tissue, regulating the amount for building of and withdrawing from bone. This dynamic homeostasis is controlled by two interbalanced regulatory agents:
    a.   vitamin and thyroid hormone
    b.   ascorbic acid and growth hormone
    c.   phosphorus and ACTH
    d.   vitamin D and parathyroid hormones

2. Phosphorus functions as a partner with calcium in building bones and teeth. Unlike calcium, however, phosphorus also plays a vital role in cell metabolism as:
    a.   an essential component for building inner cells structures
    b.   a key material in protein metabolism as a coenzyme factor in tissue synthesis
    c.   the necessary element for activating and binding processes that enable glucose to be oxidized
    d.   a detoxifying agent to rid the cell of the materials that hinder cell metabolism

3. Optimum levels of body iron are controlled at the point of absorption, interrelated with a system of transportation and storage. Which of the following statements correctly describe this iron regulating complex?
    a.   Ferric iron (Fe^{+++}), the form in foods, requires an acid medium to reduce it to ferrous iron (Fe^{++}), the form required for absorption.
    b.   Most of the iron ingested in food--about 70% to 90%--is absorbed.
    c.   Vitamin C acts as a binding and carrying agent in the transportation and storage of iron.

d. When red blood cells are destroyed, the iron used in making the hemoglobin is excreted.

4. The only known relationship of fluoride in human metabolism is with dental health. Which of the following statements correctly describe this relationship?

   a. Large amounts of fluoride produce mottled, discolored teeth.
   b. Fluoridation of public drinking water in small amounts (1 ppm) helps prevent dental caries.
   c. Topical application of fluoride solutions to young developing teeth are not effective treatment.
   d. Fluoride prevents dental caries by constructing enamel-forming organs.

Matching

Write the correct word(s) and corresponding letter in each of the numbered blanks below.

_____	1.	Chief cation guardian of the extracellular fluid
_____	2.	An ion carrying a negative electrical charge
_____	3.	Sodium-conserving mechanism or control agent
_____	4.	Simple passage of water molecules (solvent) through a membrane separating solutions of different concentrations, from the side of lower concentration of solutes to that of higher concentration of solutes, thus tending to equalize the solutions
_____	5.	A substance (atom or group of atoms) that, in solution, conducts an electric current and is dissociated into cations and anions
_____	6.	Particles, such as electrolytes and protein, in solution
_____	7.	State of dynamic equilibrium maintained by an organism among all its parts and controlled by many finely balanced mechanisms
_____	8.	Chief cation guardian of the intracellular fluid
_____	9.	Major plasma protein, which guards and maintains the circulating blood volume
_____	10.	Abnormal increase of water held in tissues
_____	11.	Any ion carrying a positive charge
_____	12.	Net filtration pressure, resulting from the difference in opposing forces of hydrostatic pressure and colloidal osmotic pressure
_____	13.	Force exerted by a contained fluid, for example, blood pressure
_____	14.	Passive movement of particles throughout a solution and across membranes from the area of denser concentration of solutes outward to all surrounding spaces
_____	15.	A part of the extracellular fluid compartment

_____ 16. Movement of solute particles in a solution across cell membranes against normal osmotic pressures, involving a second carrier substance and using a energy-dependent "pump" mechanism

_____ 17. Water-conserving mechanism, or control agent

_____ 18. Chief anion of the extracellular fluid

a. osmosis
b. solutes
c. diffusion
d. cation
e. interstitial fluid
f. homeostasis
g. anion
h. K^+
i. albumin
j. hydrostatic pressure
k. Na^+
l. electrolyte
m. active transport
n. aldosterone
o. ADH
p. capillary fluid shift mechanism
q. edema
r. Cl^-

Learning Activities

Situational Problems

Newborn feeding You are in an isolated mountain community. With the public health nurse, you visit a young mother after the delivery of her first baby. You find that the mother is feeding the newborn baby undiluted cow's milk. You notice that the baby makes jerking or twitching motions, apparently having some kind of muscle spasm.

1. On the basis of your observations and knowledge of nutritional regulatory agents so far, what do you think is causing the baby's muscle spasms?

2. What mineral balance may be involved? How is the necessary balanced ratio maintained in the body?

3. What additional information would you need to help you find some practical solutions to this problem?

4. What solutions would you propose to the mother?

Water-electrolyte imbalance An African child suffering from kwashiorkor, a protein deficiency disease, or a starving child in an urban ghetto displays a swollen abdomen filled with fluid. He grows weaker and contracts a parasitic infection; massive diarrhea follows with much sodium loss. As the diarrhea continues, increased potassium loss

84

occurs also. Finally, death occurs from cardiac arrest.

1. Account for the fluid imbalance resulting in the swollen abdomen full of fluid.
2. What causes potassium loss in prolonged diarrhea? Why is this a serious problem?
3. What causes the cardiac arrest?

Child feeding On a visit to a neighbor's home you notice that her 16-month-old child appears particularly pale, listless, and irritable. The child is taking some milk from a bottle. The mother says, "I don't understand what's wrong with her. She doesn't eat much solid food, but I see that she gets plenty of milk." You know that the father works at night and sleeps during the day. The mother has always used a bottle of formula to keep the baby from crying and disturbing him.

1. On the basis of your observations, what nutritional problem can you identify in this child?
2. What is the reason for it? Describe the role of the regulatory agent involved.
3. What solutions to the problem would you propose? Why?
4. At what other period in this child's life is this nutrient likely to be low? Why?

Community malnutrition A nurse in the Peace Corps working in central Africa visits an outlying clinic. Several of her patients, both children and adults, have enlarged thyroid glands. In one woman the gland has become so engorged that it is about the size of a grapefruit, weighing about 1 lb. It is causing her some difficulty in swallowing. The nurse realizes that treatment now would probably have little effect in reducing the fibrotic gland.

1. From this observation, what general community nutritional problem can you identify?
2. Discuss the disease process involved and what the role of the regulatory agent is in it.
3. What practical measures can you propose to control the disease in this community?
4. What additional information would you need to help you define the problem an plan your solution?

Current Nutrition Issues

Read carefully the *Issues and Answers* article "Do We Need More?: Guidelines for Trace Elements Supplementation" (*Essentials of Nutrition and Diet Therapy*, ed 6., p 163); *Nutrition and Diet Therapy*, ed 7, p 267). Consider these inquiry questions:

1. How do you account for the increased use of trace mineral supplements? How do you evaluate these practices?

2. Are there any potential dangers in use of these supplements?

3. What persons do you think may be more likely to use these supplements? Why?

4. Compare the functions, requirements, food sources, and possible toxicity of the trace elements listed here. Is a supplement of any of these warranted? If so, by whom, in what situations, and how large a dosage?

Chapter 9
THE FOOD ENVIRONMENT AND FOOD HABITS

Chapter Focus

Our rapidly changing environment is bringing changes in the needs of our clients and patients and in our own health care methods and roles. To meet this challenge, our community nutrition and health care must center on personal need, drawing not only on our special knowledge and skill but also upon our compassion and concern.

Summary-Review Quiz

Fill in the blanks below with the appropriate number and word(s) from the list following each section. Each numbered word or phrase is used; some may be used more than once. When you have completed all the sections, check your answers for each blank ny the test key (Appendix, p 257). Correct any mistakes and then review the entire chapter summary.

Food Environment

1.   An individual's state of nutrition is the direct result of the _____ of three basic factors: (1) the _____ of nutrition, which is food, (2) the _____ that receives the food, which is the person involved: and (3) the _____, which influences both food and the person involved. The study of human nutrition, based on the vast complex web formed by these three sets of interrelated forces, is spoken of as the _____ of human nutrition.

2.   The agent of malnutrition is _____. This state may be caused by a deficiency in _____, either because the total community _____ is decreased by disaster, poor distribution, or poverty, or because the person does not eat what is available.

3.   The _____, or victim, of malnutrition is the person involved. Some individual factors that may influence such a state include: (1) presence of other _____, such as infection; (2) added _____ in stress periods such as _____; (3) _____, such as prematurity or cleft palate, which influence food intake; and (4) other personal factors such as _____ of food needs or values, or the presence of _____ problems that may control food choices and appetite habits.

1. environment
2. disease
3. birth defects
4. lack of food
5. growth and pregnancy
6. agent
7. emotional
8. quantity
9. host
10. ignorance
11. interaction
12. nutrient demands
13. food supply
14. ecology

4.   Many environmental factors influence malnutrition. These factors include
_____, which produces food contamination and disease; _____ and
habits concerning food; _____ created by poverty and race; and _____,
such as rejection of a child by the mother. Also _____ problems may result
from the region's power structure. This governing structure influences the amount of
_____ an individual has to buy food in the market and controls _____
and distribution. In addition, the area's _____ determine what foods can and will
be grown.
5.   On a world level, malnutrition problems are compounded by _____ and
_____ policies. Nutritional and international _____ reveal that
malnutrition is not confined merely to _____ nations of the world. It also exists
in America because of a basic imbalance among these _____ factors and the
fundamental problem of _____.

1. psychologic problems	6. underdeveloped	11. poor sanitation
2. agricultural policies	7. cultural beliefs	12. population increase
3. poverty	8. nutrition surveys	13. food supply
4. money	9. economic and political	14. social problems
5. export/import	10. environmental	

6.   The _____ environment is a primary factor in the nutritional status of
individuals because _____ is a basic necessity for getting adequate food, and the
_____ of government programs controls food _____ and _____.
7.   Tremendous problems exist among the poor. Such _____ living
conditions breed feelings of _____ from the rest of society, _____ to
change things, and insecurity. To help meet such problems, health workers must
understand their own _____, build relationships based on mutual _____,
accept _____ as they are, and _____ carefully to each client in an open
manner.

1. availability	5. powerlessness	9. persons
2. survival	6. listen	10. distribution
3. money	7. cultural biases	11. isolation
4. respect and trust	8. economic and political	12. politics

Food Habits
1.   Food habits, as well as other aspects of any culture, are _____. This
means that we all have _____ concerning foods and their use that make up our
total _____ pattern.

2.	Food habits are _____ as part of one's culture, often s a means of _____ to the environment or _____ common natural life experiences. One's culture determines what is acceptable as _____. Our _____ and politics also influence food acceptance or rejection. Major _____, such as birth and death, coming-of-age rituals, weddings, and especially _____, are associated with special food habits and beliefs.

3.	Specific _____ have developed within different ethnic groups, built around _____ used at special events and _____, as well as everyday family meals.

4.	A key factor in the appreciation of different food patterns is a recognition of the value of _____. There can be _____ in the number and timing of meals, in the types of food used and their _____, as well as in the place food is eaten. No one way is the only "right" way. Only _____ and _____ food habits require change and then only in a _____ manner.

1. learned	7. pregnancy	13. life experiences
2. culturally acceptable	8. adapting	14. preparation
3. holidays	9. traditional foods	15. food behavior
4. human food	10. variety	16. cultural food patterns
5. harmful	11. nutritionally inadequate	17. religion
6. cultural biases	12. ethnocentric	18. interpreting

5.	Groupings of persons in a society according to family, _____, education, occupation, or residence form that society's _____. This structure influences _____, life styles, and habits. Food is closely related to _____, such as the attitude of a mother toward her maternal role, the use of certain foods to help gain _____ in one's group, or the building of close _____.

6.	The most limiting factors in determining family food choices are _____ and _____. Often displaced persons of other cultures lead a marginal existence in _____ in crowded city area. Social problems of _____ and _____ often add to poor food habits and _____ results.

1. status	5. poverty	9. wealth
2. food availability	6. social relationships	10. family relationships
3. social classes	7. family income	11. alienation
4. family structure change	8. malnutrition	12. value systems

7.	Food plays a large part in meeting basic _____. Such a hierarchy of human need is based on five progressive levels of need: _____, _____, _____, _____, and _____. Two important related factors in shaping food habits are _____, which determines personal goals, and _____, which determines how we _____ things in our environments.

8.   Foods often have _____. During illness and other stress periods, _____ to "comfort" foods, according to their _____ value, may occur.

1. comfort and security   5. love   9. psychologic needs
2. motivation   6. interpret   10. self-worth and status
3. symbolic meanings   7. self-fulfillment   11. perception
4. psychosocial   8. regression   12. physical hunger

9.   In an effort to meet human need, _____ usually based on food misinformation often develop. Persons especially susceptible to such false food claims are _____ trying to hold on to youthful vigor, _____ stretching for the competitive edge, _____ concerned with appearance, _____ burdened by social prejudices, and _____ seeking peer-acceptance.

10.   Such _____ claims usually are made for _____, rather than for _____ contained in them. No _____ controls specific body functions. People require _____, never _____. As a result of such _____ claims, a number of _____ have developed, which are contradicted by _____.

1. false   5. scientific food facts   9. specific foods
2. aging persons   6. entertainers   10. obese persons
3. specific nutrients   7. foods as such   11. food fads
4. young persons   8. food myths   12. athletes

11.   Many new _____ are adding to the problem of food choices. These new products have been developed for reasons of _____ in preparation and desire for greater _____ of food forms or for _____. The influence of mass media such as _____ creates tremendous markets for such new products, but the total impact of such advertising is often misleading and _____ in effect, especially in its influence on _____.

12.   Food additives may include _____ added as pesticides to increase crop yields and to prevent _____, or they may be substances used in _____ to produce new food forms. The _____ is the government agency responsible for controlling the use of such materials used in agriculture and the _____ and for establishing _____. This agency, together with other _____, is also mandated to maintain public _____ against food-borne disease, and to provide continuing _____ concerning food and health.

13.   As the number of new food products increases, however, problems with
_____ , such as those on the _____ list, also increase. In response to this
increased consumer concern, new regulations concerning _____ and
_____ of food products have been established under the Nutrition Labeling and
Education Act of 1990, results effective by 1993-1994.

1. FDA
2. food testing
3. convenience
4. food processing
5. food industry
6. nutrition labeling

7. antinutrition
8. processed foods
9. food spoilage
10. food additives
11. food sanitation and safety
12. television

13. agricultural chemicals
14. food standards
15. GRAS
16. fast snack foods
17. variety
18. children
19. consumer education
20. Public Health agencies

Discussion Questions

1.   What does the word "ecology" mean? How does this apply to nutrition and
       malnutrition? On this basis can you suggest any constructive approaches or
       solutions to the related problems of malnutrition?

2.   From your own observations or experiences, what economic and political factors
       influence a person's nutrition and health status? Give some examples. What
       solutions would you suggest?

3.   What basic historical values have shaped Americans' social value system? Do
       you think that some of these values are changing? Why? What effect is this
       having on food forms and habits?

4.   Define the words "motivation" and "perception," first as you find them in a
       dictionary and then in relation to food habits.

5.   Why do you think food fads develop? Cite some examples from your own
       observation or experience.

6. Why would illness or psychologic stress such as grief cause persons to regress to earlier food habits? Give some examples.

7. Is three meals a day and no snacking a basic requirement for good health and nutrition? Support your answer.

8. Describe changes you have observed in American food patterns. What factors do you think have caused these changes? What is your own general eating pattern?

9. What have been some of the major determinants of food choices and habits in your own life? Have you changed any of your eating patterns? Why? Was it easy or difficult? Why?

10. What does the phrase "a culture of poverty" mean?

11. What is the GRAS list? What problems are related to it?

Self-Test Questions

True-False
Circle the "T" if a statement is true and write a brief rationale for its accuracy. If it is false, circle the "F" and write the correct statement.

T F 1. In the United States, surveys reveal little or no real malnutrition.

T F 2. The politics of a region or county is not involved in the nutritional status of the people.

T F 3. The number of new processed food items using food additives has been declining in recent years because of public pressure and concern.

T F 4. The use of pesticides on farm crops and food additives in processed foods are under the control of the USDA and FDA.

T	**F**	5.	Food habits result from our instinctive behavioral responses throughout life.
T	**F**	6.	Social class structure in American society is largely determined by income, occupation, education, and residence.
T	**F**	7.	Life-styles change as society's values change.
T	**F**	8.	From the time of birth, eating is a social act, built on social relationships.
T	**F**	9.	High status foods usually become so because they have higher nutritional food values.
T	**F**	10.	Food fads are usually long lasting and seldom change.
T	**F**	11.	Special food combinations are effective as reducing diets and have special therapeutic effects.

Multiple Choice

Circle the letter in front of the correct answer. Then check your answers by the test key (Appendix, p 258). Now compare all the possible answers for each item and write the following brief statements: (1) rationale for the correct answer and (2) why each one of the other responses is wrong.

1. Food additives are used in processed food items to:
   (1) preserve food and lengthen its market life
   (2) enrich food with added nutrients
   (3) improve the food's general flavor, texture, or appearance
   (4) enhance or change some physical property of the food
   (5) create a new product market to meet industry competition and increase the food processor's profit
   a. 1, 4, and 5
   b. 2 and 3
   c. 1 and 5
   d. all of these
2. The use of food additives in food products is under the control of the:
   a. U.S. Public Health Department
   b. U.S. Department of Agriculture
   c. Food and Drug Administration
   d. Federal Trade Commission
3. A healthy body requires:
   a. specific foods to control specific functions
   b. certain food combinations to achieve specific physiologic effects
   c. natural foods to prevent disease
   d. specific nutrients in different foods to perform specified body functions

93

4. Food habits in a given culture are largely based on:
   (1)   food availability and agricultural development
   (2)   genetic group differences in food tastes responsible for the development of likes and dislikes
   (3)   food economics, market practices, and food distribution
   (4)   symbolic meanings attached to certain foods
   a.   1, 2, and 3
   b.   1, 3, and 4
   c.   1 and 3 only
   d.   all of these

5. In the Jewish food pattern, the word *kosher* refers to food that is prepared by:
   (1)   ritual slaughter of allowed animals with maximum blood drainage
   (2)   avoiding meat and milk combinations in the same meal
   (3)   special seasonings to avoid salt use
   (4)   special methods of cooking food combinations to ensure their purity and digestibility
   a.   1 and 3
   b.   2 and 4
   c.   1 and 2
   d.   3 and 4

6. Stir-frying is a method of cooking vegetables used in the food pattern of:
   a.   Mexican-Americans
   b.   Chinese
   c.   Jews
   d.   Greeks

7. The basic grain used in the Mexican food patterns is:
   a.   rice
   b.   corn
   c.   wheat
   d.   oat

8. In working with patients of different cultural food habits, what principles should guide the health worker in helping them meet their nutritional needs?
   (1)   Learn as much as possible about the person's cultural habits related to nutrition and health.
   (2)   Analyze findings in an unprejudiced manner on the basis of known nutritional science and local conditions
   (3)   Encourage traditional practices that are beneficial.
   (4)   Do not interfere with practices that are harmless.
   (5)   Try to overcome harmful practices by persuasion and demonstration.
   a.   1, 2, and 5 only
   b.   2, 3, and 4 only
   c.   all of the above
   d.   1 and 5 only

Learning Activities

Individual Survey: Food Labeling—Additives and Nutrients

Visit a local community food market and survey the variety of food products. Find as many new processed food items as you can, at least ten. Read the label on each one carefully and study the nature and use of the item.

1. List the food items that you located. Describe each in terms of its general nature, packaging, and use.
2. What does the label on each item tell you about how the food was processed? List the food additives used and determine the purpose of as many of them as you can. Call your nearest FDA district office for information or write to the Federal office in Washington, D.C., for information on food additives.
3. Did you find information on the labels about nutrient values or other nutrition information about the food items? Give examples.
4. How would you evaluate these processed food items?

Individual Survey: Cultural Food Patterns

Select a person of a different cultural background from your own and interview this person concerning food habits. Use the food groupings given in Tool A (p 295) to inquire about food items most commonly used and general methods of preparing them. Then ask about the basic meal pattern for a day, filling in the form in Tool B (p 296). Compare your findings with the discussion of this cultural food pattern in your textbook and other resources.

Group Project: International Food Festival

Plan an international dinner with your class by having students with different cultural backgrounds prepare some of their ethnic dishes and describe their use and preparation in their culture. Other students may select any additional ethnic foods that they wish to provide for the dinner.

Prepare an exhibit table of cookbooks for different types of ethnic cooking, special cooking and eating utensils, special seasonings, unusual foods or pictures of foods, and any other cultural artifacts related to food.

Invite any other persons that you may know from different cultures to present some of their foods.

Your may wish to collect some of the group's favorite recipes and prepare copies in a booklet for each person to have.

Current Nutritional Issues

Read carefully the *Issues and Answers* article "The Spice of Ethnic Diversity in American Food Patterns" (*Essentials of Nutrition and Diet Therapy*, ed 6, p 189; *Nutrition and Diet Therapy*, ed 7, p 316). Consider these inquiry questions:

1. Give some examples of how religious laws govern Jewish and Moslem food patterns. Describe any ways you see here that food is used not only for nourishment but also for teaching purposes.

2. What personal and cultural values do you think the current blending of a variety of cultural food patterns is contributing to American culture?

3. How does our own American history show up in our various regional food patterns? Describe these roots and the developing food pattern for several of our regional food habits, using examples to illustrate, perhaps from your own family food patterns.

Chapter 10
FAMILY NUTRITION COUNSELING: FOOD NEEDS AND COSTS

Chapter Focus

Person-centered, goal-directed counseling is a fundamental component of all health care, especially nutritional care. To be realistic, related teaching-learning activities must actively involve the human personality, valid principles of learning, and appropriate resources to help meet identified personal needs.

Summary-Review Quiz

Fill in the blanks below with the appropriate number and word(s) from the list following each section. Each numbered word or phrase is used; some may be used more than once. When you have completed all the sections, check your answers for each blank by the test key (Appendix, p 259). Correct any mistakes and then review the entire chapter summary.

1.   The basic goal of health care is to help individuals meet their _____. To achieve this goal, three types of health care activities are fundamental: (1) obtaining basic _____ about the _____ and the _____ that relates to _____, (2) providing health _____ to help meet these _____, and (3) providing _____ for efforts to meet _____, through general encouragement and _____.

2.   Skills in _____ are basic to any nutritional care plan. This activity may be a structured _____ to obtain a _____, but often it is a more formal goal-directed _____. The _____ is always on the patient or client and individual _____. The _____ is always to provide whatever _____ is required to meet personal _____ and goals.

1. support	6. purpose	11. health needs
2. interview	7. information	12. planned conversation
3. living situation	8. diet history	13. positive reinforcement
4. focus	9. teaching	14. individual patient or client
5. interviewing	10. help	

3.   The health worker's means of accomplishing this basic purpose include: (1) a trustful _____, (2) a comfortable _____, and (3) attitudes of _____ showing genuine concern, _____ (taking persons as they are), _____ (avoiding bias), and _____ (feeling with clients and patients).

4.   During the interview, the health worker must _____ physical features and behavior patterns, _____ carefully to understand what is being said and _____ in appropriate words or gestures. Some means of _____ the interview's main points should be planned.

1. acceptance	5. compassion	9. observe
2. listen	6. objectivity	10. warmth
3. respond	7. recording	
4. climate	8. relationship	

5.   Several means may be used to obtain a _____: (1) _____, in which patients describe their food intake during the previous day; (2) _____, on which patients may check how often they use key food items; (3)_____, which patients may keep for 3 to 7 days or longer; and (4)_____ food habits interview, in which patients relate general daily food use to daily routines.

6.   The food intake is then _____ with the client or patient to determine _____ and any individual food-related _____ involved. Using these _____ as a guide, _____ can be determined. Then a personal _____ is developed. Follow-up _____ is needed to plan any necessary _____.

7.   A _____ program may follow initial _____ of learning needs, with _____ learning activities planned to meet _____. In addition, _____ and discussion may help provide _____ from other patients as well, to help make wise self-care decisions.

1. analyzed	7. nutrition education	13. nutrition history
2. identified needs	8. problems	14. assessment
3. food records	9. support	15. goals for care
4. individual	10. activity-associated	16. group instruction
5. evaluation	11. food plan	17. food frequency lists
6. 24-hour recall	12. modifications	18. nutritional needs

8.   Suggestions for _____ can help persons spend limited food dollars more wisely. Careful _____ will help prevent wasteful food spoilage. Government food assistance programs such as the _____ for low-income families of the _____ for needy families may be required.

9.   The _____ is a government food aid program for _____ agricultural surpluses to help provide a _____ for farm products. Therefore, because its primary objective is to support _____, it does not totally meet _____ of _____ persons. The number, form, and variety of the foods available often provides _____. Its mode of _____ is often unusable. Its method of _____ presents problems for some disabled, ill, or _____ persons to get the food and carry it home. Also the _____ built into the program's administrative barriers turns many needy people off.

1. Food Stamp Program
2. poor
3. price support
4. packaging
5. storage of food
6. elderly
7. nutritional needs
8. social stigma
9. Commodities Distribution Program
10. inadequate nutrition
11. economy buying
12. distribution
13. farm prices
14. buying and storing

10. The _____ offers food assistance by extending the buying power of a poor person's _____. Monthly _____ are distributed to participating _____. Eligibility is based on _____ and the limit is quite _____, so participating families just don't make enough _____ to buy _____.

11. The _____ provides _____ to schools to provide meals for _____ students. Poor children can eat _____ and other students pay _____. Participating schools receive _____. Lunches served must meet _____ of the child's _____ for nutrients. Because the program is under local school control, however, its administration has often been hindered by _____ and _____. The recently enacted Child Nutrition Act has liberalized the program to include _____ children and a _____ meal.

1. households
2. food
3. all
4. one third
5. food dollar
6. local prejudice
7. School Lunch Program
8. reduced rates
9. preschool
10. low
11. food coupons
12. financial assistance
13. lack of funds
14. Food Stamp Program
15. breakfast
16. commodity foods
17. gross income
18. RDA
19. free meals
20. money

Discussion Questions

1. What is meant by the *climate* of the interview? Describe some ways that you as a health worker may help your patient or client feel comfortable. Be as specific as you can with examples.

2. Compare the various ways of obtaining a diet history. How would you use each to secure valid and useful information? What would you then do with this information?

99

3. Why is information about the individual life situation important in planning nutritional care and education? How would you involve the patient or client in this planning process?

4. Why is the manner of terminating an interview important? Suggest several constructive ways that this may be done.

5. What responsibility does the health worker have regarding the patient's or client's chart?

6. Give some realistic suggestions that you might use in diet counseling with a low-income family.

Self-Test Questions

<u>True-False</u>
Circle the "T" if a statement is true and write a brief rationale for its accuracy. If it is false, circle the "F" and write the correct statement.

T F 1. Attitudes are learned from total life experience and form the basis of behavior.
T F 2. The human brain can assimilate and interpret all the information that the senses take in.
T F 3. The average person has only about 25% listening efficiency.
T F 4. More accurate food records usually result when the patient is given reasons for keeping them and the specific type of information needed.
T F 5. The tougher, less expensive cuts of meat have less food value.
T F 6. The shell color of eggs affects their quality and food value.
T F 7. Nonfat milk has less protein value than whole milk.
T F 8. Fruits and vegetables are the main sources of vitamins A and C.
T F 9. Higher grades of canned fruits and vegetables have higher food values.
T F 10. Enriched and whole grain cereals and breads are usually nutrition bargains.

<u>Multiple Choice</u>

Circle the letter in front of the correct answer. Then check your answers by the test key (Appendix, p 260). Now compare all the possible answers for each item and write the following brief statements: (1) rationale for the correct answer and (2) why each one of the other responses is wrong.

1. The purpose of the health worker is to help patients meet individual health needs. This purpose can best be achieved by which of the following actions?
    (1)   Encourage patients to talk about their ideas, feelings, and desires for their own care.
    (2)   Assure them that the staff is well qualified and will attend to all of their needs.
    (3)   Tell them that decisions about their care will be made for them, so that they can relax and need ask no questions.
    (4)   Discuss with patients helpful information about possible ways of meeting their care needs and let them help plan solutions.
    a.   1 and 4
    b.   2 and 3
    c.   1 and 2
    d.   3 and 4

2. Acceptance of patients means:
    (1)   constant approval of their behavior
    (2)   viewing their behavior as purposeful to them
    (3)   believing that their actions are worth attention
    (4)   valuing their worth as persons
    a.   1, 3, and 4
    b.   all of these
    c.   2, 3, and 4
    d.   1, 2, and 4

3. The art of listening requires careful attention to:
    (1)   words that the patient uses and repetition of key words
    (2)   tone of voice and feelings expressed
    (3)   the overall content of what is being said
    (4)   silences and being comfortable with them
    a.   1 and 3
    b.   2 and 3
    c.   2 and 4
    d.   all of these

4. Responses to the patient during the interview may be in the form of:
   (1)   silence, touch, or gesture
   (2)   clear unbiased questions
   (3)   restatements of the patient's own statements
   (4)   reflection of expressed feelings
   a.   2 and 3
   b.   all of these
   c.   3 and 4
   d.   1 and 4
5. Specific charting requirements will vary in different health care facilities. However, after a clinic interview with a patient, certain types of information should be recorded in the chart. Which of the following might this include?
   (1)   general description of the patient's physical status
   (2)   appropriate observations concerning emotional state or expressed attitudes and concerns
   (3)   description of care or teaching provided and the results
   (4)   plans for follow-up appointments or visits
   a.   1 and 3
   b.   2 and 4
   c.   all of these
   d.   2 and 3
6. Which of the following interview statements would be most likely to obtain accurate information concerning a patient's breakfast habits?
   a.   "Do you always eat breakfast every morning?"
   b.   "Breakfast skipping is a bad habit."
   c.   "Everyone should always start the day with a good breakfast."
   d.   "After you get up in the morning, if you have something to eat, what might it be?"
7. Which of the following statements would be most helpful in obtaining accurate information about a patient's use of milk?
   a.   "Do you drink plenty of milk?"
   b.   "Everybody needs milk."
   c.   "Do you mean you drink only a glass of milk a day?"
   d.   "You mentioned having milk at dinner. Would you say then that you usually have about one glass a day?

Learning Activities

Individual Interview: Nutrition History and Analysis
    Using Tool A (p 297) and Tool B (p 298), interview any selected individual to obtain a nutrition history. Make a basic nutritional analysis of the person's food intake by comparing it with the generally used food groups.
   1.   What actions or responses did you observe during the interview concerning this person's attitudes toward food and nutrition?

2.   What were your own feelings during the interview? Were you comfortable in your role of interviewer?

3.   Did you and the person make the nutritional analysis together, or did you do it yourself later?

4.   Which analysis action do you think may be more useful to the person?

5.   What was the result of your analysis? Were there any deficiencies you could generally detect?

6.   What suggestions, if any, did you make to the person that would improve the diet? What could you have suggested in the light of your findings?

Group Project: Interview Recordings and Analysis

For students involved in patient or client care in any type of health care setting, an analysis of the interviewing process is helpful in developing the ability to *hear* and *understand* what the patient is really saying. Many clues may be detected in communication from the patient and in your responses to help identify real needs. Also, facilitating or hindering responses may be identified.

Materials   Tape recorder, or video tape equipment if available, and clients or patients in home, hospital, or clinic settings.

Procedure

1.   Using the history interview guides in your textbook, have several students conduct individual interviews with selected patients concerning food habits.

2.   Secure the patient's permission to tape record the interview, giving assurances of privacy and use of the tape only for learning purposes.

3.   Conduct the interview as discussed above.

4.   As a group, with instructor guidance as needed, develop a guide for analyzing the interviews.

5.   Listen or view the tapes as a group, with each student marking an evaluation guidesheet for each interview.

6.   Discuss the interviews according to the evaluation points on the guidesheet.

Results

1.   List the main points of the analysis guide developed by your group.

2.   How did the interviews compare, according to these evaluation points?

Discussions

1.   What strong points did you identify in these recorded interviews? What do you consider their strength to be?

2. What weak points did you identify? What suggestions can you make for their improvement?

Class Experiment: Observation Skills
Procedure
1. Divide the class into small groups of two or three members each.
2. Have each group visit a different public place, such as several blocks of a downtown area, an airport or clinic waiting room, or a public restaurant.
3. Each group member is to take notes concerning observations made during the activity, but no discussion of observations or comparison of notes is to be done.
4. In the following class meeting, each group member is to present to the rest of the class a list of individual observations.

Results
1. What common observations were reported by all group members?

2. What observations were reported by only one person?

Discussion
1. What determines what a person *sees*?

2. Can you account for these specific similarities and differences in the observations made by each member of your group?

Group Experiment: Listening Skills
Another means of developing skills in communication, especially in listening and clarifying meaning, has been used in a variety of adaptations. In situations involving groups of 10 to 15 students, the students work in pairs in a role-playing type of situation.
Procedure
1. Assign a role and situation to one of the partners without the knowledge of the other.

2. Bring the two students together and have the person with the assigned role (for example, that of a patient in a clinical setting with a health problem) initiate the conversation.

3. As the two talk together, the second student is to play the role of the health worker. She may communicate only by making responses to statements made by the first student playing the role of the patient. Her purpose is to clarify meaning through restatement of reflective responses and relevant questions until she can state the patient's position and problem to his situation as he sees it.

4. If at any point the student playing the role of the health worker interjects irrelevant statements or material or personal comments, the group is to interrupt and call this to the attention of the student playing the health worker.

5. Resume the interaction until the patient's problem is fully identified and clarified to his satisfaction.

Results

1. List the number of times the conversation had to be interrupted by the group because the student acting as the health worker did not hear an important clue given by the student playing the role of the patient.

2. List those clues given by the patient that were picked up and responded to by the health worker.

Discussion

1. What barriers to communication are frequently used in conversation?

2. Give some types of responses that would help a person to clarify his meaning.

3. What does the term *creative listening* mean to you? What is its basic purpose?

Individual Project: Market Survey of Comparative Foods Costs

Procedure

1. Select ten food items that may be marketed in different forms.
2. Visit a local community market and compare the different forms in which you find each food item—for example, frozen, fresh, canned, processed.
3. List the price that you find for each form of the item and the amount of food in that market unit.

Results

1. List each of the food items that you located and the unit price for each form.

2. What form generally was the least expensive?

Discussion

1. In view of your finding, what suggestions can you give for economical food buying?

2. What factors influence the cost of food items?

Group Project: Food Economics and a Welfare Budget for a Family of Four

Problem How can a family of four persons living on a welfare allowance meet their nutritional requirements?

Materials Current price information on foods from a variety of community food outlets, information concerning food assistance programs in the community, and food value tables and recommended dietary allowances (RDA) of nutrients (textbook).

Procedure

1. Consider carefully the following family of four: father, age 27, disabled and unable to work; a mother, age 25; and two children--a boy, age 9, and a girl, age 5. At present the family has five members because the grandmother is staying with them indefinitely. The are on welfare and receive from the state the equivalent of 18 cents per person per day for a food allowance. (State welfare allowances for food vary widely. To make this project more realistic, if possible, find out this family's welfare allowance for food in your state and use that figure per person per day in your project.)

2. Make a tentative food plan for one week for the family, using generally low-cost food items. From this week's menu, make out a market list for shopping.

3. Divide your group and assign different members to different stores of the following types to price the foods on your list:
   regular supermarket
   small neighborhood grocery store
   community food cooperative
   farmer's market
   damaged goods store (dented or unlabeled cans, etc.)
   natural food store

4. From your comparative shopping survey, select the best food items and calculate the cost per serving.

5. Revise your original menu as needed, according to the food prices you found. Using your welfare money allowance for a day's food for five persons, calculate the cost of 1 day's food for this family.

6. Check the nutritional adequacy of this day's menu for one family member, for example, the father. First, calculate the food values in your diet plan, using the food value tables in your textbook, Appendix A. Then compare your totals for each nutrient with the recommended dietary allowance for the nutrient.

7. Investigate the available food assistance programs in the community. Interview by phone or in person a representative in your local welfare office or public health office. Secure any printed materials or guides that may be available.

Results

1. Of the food buying sources you surveyed, where did you find the best buys? How did the cost of your listed food items compare in the various types of stores?

2. Describe your experience with the welfare office in trying to secure information about welfare food allowances.

3. What food assistance programs operate in your community? What attitudes did you discover toward persons using these programs?

107

4. Within your limited food cost allowance, what nutrients did you find the most difficult in securing in adequate amounts? How did your nutrient calculations compare with the recommended dietary allowances for each nutrient?

Discussion

1. From your findings, what solutions can you suggest for this family to help them meet their nutritional needs within their limited financial circumstances?

2. What do you think your role may be in helping to meet the basic nutritional needs of poverty families—as (a) a health worker or (b) a public citizen?

3. Is any national or state legislation under study for changes in these food-related programs?

Current Nutritional Issues

Read carefully the *To Probe Further* box, "Effect of Adult Learning Concepts on the Nutrition Interview" (*Essentials of Nutrition and Diet Therapy*, ed 6, p 200); *Nutrition and Diet Therapy*, ed 7, p 325); and the *Issues and Answers* article, "A Person-Centered Model Applied to Diabetes Education" (*Essentials of Nutrition and Diet Therapy*, ed 6, p 208); *Nutrition and Diet Therapy*, ed 7, P 336). Consider these inquiry questions.

1. Why do you think it is important to base adult education and counseling programs on personal attitudes and tested learning theories?

2. Give some examples to support your answer to the question above.

3. In relation to the effectiveness of a learning process, what does the term "psychological safety" mean to you? Apply this meaning to a counseling or learning experience of your own.

4. Can you give examples in patient education in which good self-care, and hence the learning process, is especially important to a person with a particular health problem?

Chapter 11
NUTRITION DURING PREGNANCY AND LACTATION

Chapter Focus

Sound nutritional support largely determines the successful outcome of a woman's pregnancy. The normal healthy growth and development of both mother and baby relate directly to the good diet of the mother.

Summary-Review Quiz

Fill in the blanks below with the appropriate number and word(s) from the list following each section. Each numbered word or phrase is used; some may be used more than once. When you have completed all the sections, check your answers for each blank by the test key (Appendix, p 261). Correct any mistakes and then review the entire chapter summary.

1. Much of the nutritional advice given to prenatal patients in American obstetric practice in the past has been based on _____, not _____. As a result, two _____ grew and governed practice: (1) the _____ (whatever the fetus needs it will draw from the mother, no matter how deficient her diet), and (2) the _____ (whatever the fetus needs, the mother will crave and consume).

2. Today scientific evidence for the _____ of pregnancy is overwhelming. These nutritional needs during pregnancy are determined by three basic factors: (1) the _____ of the mother, (2) her _____ state of nutrition, and (3) the complex _____ of gestation. The interdependent biologic functions of _____, _____ and _____ during a pregnancy form a unique biologic _____, a good example of physiologic _____.

1. increased nutritional demands
2. metabolic interactions
3. parasite theory
4. fetus
5. scientific fact
6. synergism
7. age and parity
8. placenta
9. maternal instinct theory
10. whole
11. mother
12. traditional assumptions
13. preconception
14. false theories

3.   Current practice in nutritional care of pregnant women supports the _____ approach of _____ to meet the increased nutritional demand. This practice refutes the past traditional _____ approach, which emphasized _____ and _____. Current guidelines provide health workers and _____ with both _____ for good prenatal care and sound _____ for good prenatal diet.

4.   Healthy women produce _____ babies within a _____ range of _____. Diets that are _____ in kcalories and _____ should be avoided because they are _____.

1. restrictive
2. optimal full diet
3. principles of nutrition
4. harmful
5. salt restriction

6. wide
7. mothers
8. healthy
9. low
10. positive

11. sodium
12. total weight gain
13. food plans
14. weight control

5.   Instead of restrictions the emphasis should be on promoting sufficient _____ to support the increased _____. Of primary concern is the _____ of the _____ and the _____ in the diet producing it, not on a specific _____, or amount, of gain.

6.   Sufficient _____ are critical to meet needs for the _____ development of extra maternal _____. This provides the necessary _____ essential for (1) rapid _____ and _____ required for delivery and _____ and (2) the _____ demand of the increased _____ of _____.

1. quality
2. adipose fat tissue
3. kilocalories
4. fetal growth
5. metabolic work

6. total weight gain
7. lactation
8. energy
9. nutrients
10. gestation

11. normal
12. metabolic demands
13. fuel storage
14. quantity

7.   A positive, sound diet for pregnancy should include increased amounts of _____ for growth. The pregnant woman needs about 60 g/day, or an increase of about _____ over her usual intake. Primary foods of _____ include _____, _____, _____, and _____. Additional secondary sources include _____ and _____.

8. Also the increased _____ for _____ will spare _____ for its building function. Active or _____ women may easily require 2500 to 3000 kcal/day.

1. complete protein   6. milk   11. high-quality protein
2. meat   7. whole or enriched grains   12. legumes
3. kilocalories   8. cheese   13. nutritionally deficient
4. 10-15 g/day   9. egg
5. protein   10. energy

9. A mineral especially needed in increased amounts is _____ for bone building. The major food sources of this major mineral are _____. Thus they should be _____ in the diet.

10. Another mineral needed is _____ because of the increased blood _____ and the added need for storage in the baby's developing _____. This storage is necessary because _____, the infant's first food, lacks _____. Without sufficient amounts of this essential trace element, _____ will develop. Food sources, however, are_____ and _____ are highly possible. For this reason a daily increase of _____ is needed. The best food source is _____. Additional sources having small amounts of this key mineral include _____, dried beans, dried fruit, _____, _____, and _____.

1. milk   6. eggs   11. anemia
2. iron   7. liver   12. meat
3. green vegetables   8. not widespread   13. calcium
4. dairy products   9. increased   14. volume
5. deficiencies   10. enriched breads and cereals

11. Increased amounts of vitamins are also required by the pregnant woman. For example, _____ is needed for epithelial tissue growth, tooth bud development, and _____. It is supplied in the diet by _____, egg yolk, and _____ or fortified _____. Major plant sources are _____ vegetables and fruits. An excess of _____, however, can cause fetal damage and must be avoided.

12. The _____ vitamin group is needed for _____ to aid in energy production and to regulate many _____. The _____ is always increased during pregnancy. A particular B-complex vitamin needed is _____ to protect against a particular kind of anemia, so a _____ is recommended.

1. B-complex   5. bone growth   9. vitamin A
2. metabolic activities 6. green and yellow 10. BMR
3. butter   7. margarine   11. coenzyme factors
4. folate   8. daily increase   12. liver

112

13.   A vitamin especially needed for tissue growth is _____. It deposits a _____ substance to help build strong tissue. A main source is _____. Other food sources include _____, potatoes, melons, _____, cabbage, and other greens.

14.   Additional _____ is needed for the absorption and use of _____ and _____, the major minerals required for bone formation. The recommended daily amount of this vitamin is _____. The main food source is _____.

1. citrus fruits	5. cementing	9. calcium
2. phosphorus	6. 10 μg cholecalciferol	10. tomatoes
3. vitamin D	7. vitamin C	
4. berries	8. fortified milk	

15.   Functional gastrointestinal _____ may occur during pregnancy. These include early _____ or later _____ as the baby enlarges. Simple dietary adjustments in _____ or _____ usually remedy this situation.

16.   A nutrition-related common complication of pregnancy is _____. The _____ of a single normal pregnancy is large, so the risk of _____ is common and a daily increase of _____ if required. A less common condition, _____ of pregnancy, results from _____, so daily increase of _____ is also needed.

1. type of food	5. nausea and vomiting	9. problems
2. iron deficiency anemia	6. iron cost	10. deficiency
3. folate	7. folate deficiency	11. meal pattern
4. iron	8. megaloblastic anemia	12. constipation

17.   A far less common but more serious complication is _____, formerly called _____, occurring in late pregnancy. It is closely associated with _____, _____, and lack of _____. It affects primarily the body's major metabolic organ, the _____. Blood levels of _____ are low. Blood _____ also decreases. Therefore diet therapy for both prevention and treatment centers on increased _____ because of the role of _____ in maintaining the circulating blood _____. The diet should not be _____ because (1) _____ is a needed _____ in the increased circulating blood _____ and (2) the root cause of the edema is the low level of _____ related to dietary _____ deficiency, not _____ use.

1. malnutrition	6. prenatal care	11. sodium
2. plasma protein	7. salt	12. pregnancy-induced hypertension (PIH)
3. salt-free	8. liver	13. poverty
4. toxemia	9. high-quality protein	14. electrolyte
5. protein	10. volume	

18. After delivery, for the breast-feeding mother, the _____ for _____ increase to provide nutrients for _____ and energy for _____. The mother's diet should provide about _____ . ___. In addition to solid foods, more _____ are also required. Exclusive_____ by well-nourished mothers can be entirely _____ for younger infant needs. Usually _____ are added to the baby's diet at the _____ of age.

1. milk production
2. adequate
3. lactation
4. 6 months

5. breast-feeding
6. fluids
7. solid foods
8. nutritional demands

9. 2500 to 2700 kcalories
10. milk content

Discussion Questions

1. Describe the role of protein in maternal nutrition in (1) the growth process involved and (2) regulation of body fluids.

2. Why are low-caloric and salt-free diets for weight control during pregnancy dangerous?

3. Why is anemia a common finding during pregnancy? What specific nutrients are needed to prevent it, and how do they function?

4. Why are the liver and its functions so important during pregnancy?

5. What does the word *synergism* mean? What is the significance of this concept in pregnancy?

6. What is the significance of the *perinatal* concept in the health of mothers and babies? What role would nutrition have in this approach?

7.   Identify risk factors involved in pregnancy and describe special counseling needs for these high-risk mothers. What damaging personal and social habits must be avoided? In each case, what is the danger involved?

Self-Test Questions

True-False

Circle the "T" if a statement is true and write a brief rationale for its accuracy. If it is false, circle the "F" and write the correct statement.

T F 1. The development of the fetus is directly related to the diet of the mother.
T F 2. The fetus will draw what it needs from the stores of the mother, despite the maternal diet.
T F 3. The mother will instinctively crave and consume whatever the fetus needs.
T F 4. Strict weight control during pregnancy is needed to avoid complications.
T F 5. Salt should be removed from the diet during pregnancy to control edema.
T F 6. A higher risk of pregnancy complications occur in teen-aged and older-age women.
T F 7. A woman's diet prior to her pregnancy has little effect on the outcome of her pregnancy.
T F 8. Physiologic generalized edema of pregnancy is a normal protective body response.
T F 9. No woman should ever gain more than 15 to 20 pounds during her pregnancy.
T F 10. The rapid growth of fetal skeletal tissue during pregnancy requires an increased intake of calcium in the maternal diet.
T F 11. Anemia is common during pregnancy because the iron requirements are increased.
T F 12. Failure to meet increased vitamin C needs during pregnancy may lead to weakened tissue formation and bleeding tendencies.
T F 13. Inadequate vitamin D during pregnancy contributes to faulty skeletal tissue development in the fetus.
T F 14. Megaloblastic anemia of pregnancy results from iron deficiency.
T F 15. Additional fluid intake is needed during lactation.

Multiple Choice

Circle the letter in front of the correct answer. Then check your answers by the test key (Appendix, p 262). Now compare all the possible answers for each item and write the following brief statements: (1) rationale for the correct answer and (2) why each one of the other responses is wrong.

115

1. To ensure sound nutrition, the mother's diet during pregnancy should include:
   (1)   Increased protein of high biologic value
   (2)   Increased kilocalories to meet increased metabolic needs
   (3)   Enough salt to maintain electrolyte balance
   (4)   Sufficient vitamins and minerals to regulate increased metabolism
   a.   1 and 2
   b.   all of these
   c.   3 and 4
   d.   1 and 4
2. *Biologic synergism* among several separate biologic entities means that:
   a.   each component acts individually and is not influenced by the others
   b.   one component is primary and the others feed on it
   c.   no interrelationship exists among the components in their metabolic functions
   d.   the constant interdependent action produces a total result greater than and different from the sum of their parts
3. Blood volume during pregnancy:
   a.   increases
   b.   decreases
   c.   remains unchanged
   d.   fluctuates widely
4. Which of the following items are necessary tissue increases during a normal pregnancy and hence account for healthy weight increase?
   (1)   fetal tissue growth
   (2)   placenta development
   (3)   maternal breast and uterus growth
   (4)   blood volume and amniotic fluid
   (5)   maternal adipose fat tissue
   a.   1, 2, 3, and 4
   b.   1, 2, 3, and 5
   c.   1, 2, and 4
   d.   all of these
5. Which of the following foods are complete proteins of high biologic value and therefore should be increased during pregnancy?
   a.   enriched whole grains and breads
   b.   milk, egg, and cheese
   c.   beans, peas, lentils
   d.   nuts, and seeds

6. Increased iron requirements during pregnancy related directly to the:
   (1) increased book volume and need for hemoglobin
   (2) storage of iron in the fetal liver
   (3) increased fetal bone formation
   (4) loss of iron in menstruation
   a. 1 and 3
   b. 2 and 4
   c. 1 and 2
   d. 3 and 4
7. The food having the highest iron content is:
   a. lean beef
   b. liver
   c. orange juice
   d. milk
8. The increased need for vitamin A during pregnancy may be met by increased use of such foods as:
   a. nonfat milk
   b. extra egg whites
   c. citrus fruits
   d. carrots
9. Which of the following diet modifications would you recommend for a woman suffering from nausea and vomiting during the early period of her pregnancy?
   (1) increased fat content
   (2) no snacks between meals
   (3) liquids used only between, rather than with, meals
   (4) frequent small meals and snacks instead of regular full meals
   (5) increased carbohydrate foods
   a. 1, 3, and 4
   b. 2, 4, and 5
   c. 3, 4, and 5
   d. 1, 2, and 3
10. What advice would you give a pregnant woman who complained of constipation in last trimester of pregnancy?
    (1) decrease fluid intake
    (2) use mild laxatives regularly
    (3) increase fluid intake
    (4) increase foods such as whole grains and dried fruits
    a. 1 and 4
    b. 2 and 3
    c. 1 and 2
    d. 3 and 4

11. Pregnancy-induced hypertension is a complication of late pregnancy characterized by:
   (1)   increased blood pressure
   (2)   increased edema and decreased blood volume
   (3)   protein i the urine and decreased serum protein
   (4)   convulsions in severe cases
   a.   1 and 4
   b.   1 and 3
   c.   all of these
   d.   1 and 2
12. Pregnancy-induces hypertension is closely related to:
   a.   malnutrition and poverty
   b.   dietary salt use
   c.   increased protein in the diet
   d.   increased carbohydrate in the diet
13. Prevention and treatment of pregnancy-induced hypertension would include which of the following recommendations?
   (1)   optimal amount of protein to increase serum protein and restore circulating blood volume
   (2)   elimination of salt to control edema
   (3)   sufficient kcalories to meet energy demands and spare protein for tissue needs
   (4)   decrease fluid intake to balance tissue fluid retention
   a.   1 and 2
   b.   3 and 4
   c.   1 and 3
   d.   2 and 4

Learning Activities

Individual Project: Nutritional analysis of Pregnant Woman's Diet

Using the general guides in your textbook, interview a pregnant woman to learn about her food habits and environment.

Calculate her intake of the following key nutrients: protein, calcium, iron, vitamin A, and vitamin C, as well as her total energy (kcalories) intake. Analyze your findings in terms of her pregnancy requirements.

Using the information gained in your interview about her living and family situation and her food habits, plan with her a suitable daily food pattern to meet her increased nutritional needs during pregnancy.

Group Project: Teaching Pregnant Women About Nutritional Needs

In a selected clinic or community setting, arrange with the staff to conduct one or more discussions with a group of pregnant women. Plan the class sessions to include the following:

1. Exploration of present notions about food needs during pregnancy and questions about the role of nutrition in pregnancy.
2. Relation of key nutrients to normal growth and development during pregnancy.
3. Food sources of each key nutrient and a basic daily food plan to meet these nutritional demands within individual cultural food patterns.
4. Evaluation of follow-up diets of each group member if possible.

Prepare a series of visual aids to demonstrate or visualize each point of your discussion. If possible, bring actual foods to use in setting up a model food plan.

Individual or Group Project: Cultural Food Pattern in Pregnancy

Select any one of the various cultural food patterns. Plan a prenatal diet within this pattern to meet the increased nutritional demands of pregnancy.

If possible, interview a pregnant woman of this cultural group and analyze her diet.

Individual or Group Project: Diet for Lactation

Interview a breast-feeding mother of a newborn baby to determine her food habits and questions concerning a diet for lactation. Discuss with her the lactation process and assist her with techniques for successful breast-feeding.

Current Nutrition Issues

Read carefully the *To Probe Further* box, "Breast-Feeding: The Dynamic Nature of Human Milk" (*Essentials of Nutrition and Diet Therapy*, ed 6., p 224; *Nutrition and Diet Therapy*, ed 7, p 360). Consider these inquiry questions:

1. Why would it not be wise for a breast-feeding mother to give added formula, juices, or semisolid foods to her 2-week-old infant?

2. Can the mother of a preterm infant successfully breast-feed baby? How is preterm human milk different?

3. How does the nature of human milk adjust when solid foods are added to the baby's diet at about 6 months of age?

4. If the mother has a cesarean section, can she still breast-feed her baby?

Chapter 12
NUTRITION FOR GROWTH AND DEVELOPMENT

Chapter Focus

Throughout the childhood years, human maturation involves both physical growth and psychosocial development. Feeding practices and food habits in each age group are intimately related to the whole integrated human process of normal growth and development--of "growing up" in any culture.

Summary-Review Quiz

Fill in the blanks below with the appropriate number and word(s) from the list following each section. Each numbered word or phrase is used; some may be used more than once. When you've completed all the sections, check your answers for each blank by the test key (Appendix, p 263). Correct any mistakes and then review the entire chapter summary.

1.   The normal human life cycle follows four general growth periods: (a) The infant grows _____ during the first year of life; at 6 months birth weight will have _____, and at 1 year it will have _____. (b) During childhood between infancy and adolescence, the growth rate _____ and becomes _____. (c) During adolescence another _____ growth rate occurs; body changes and sex characteristics develop because of the _____ influences of _____. (d) In adulthood, growth _____ and then gradually _____ in old age.

2.   The important consideration in the growth of children is that they are _____. Normal physical growth can _____.

1. rapid	5. levels off	9. rapidly
2. puberty	6. doubled	10. hormonal
3. slows	7. irregular	11. individuals
4. vary widely	8. declines	12. tripled

3.   A commonly used index to measure physical growth is _____. Other body measurements include _____ thickness, _____, and from these two measures the derived value for _____. In infant care, the _____ circumference is used. Clinical signs of growth and development can be identified from general _____ of physical and nutritional status. These signs include the condition of the oral tissues, _____; posture and vitality; condition of the _____, hair, and eyes; degree of _____ development; and _____ control. Additional laboratory measures may include _____ and _____ tests to determine levels of _____, vitamins, or various metabolites. Bone development may be determined by taking _____ of the hand and wrist.

120

1. head
2. gums and teeth
3. nervous
4. skinfold
5. hemoglobin

6. blood
7. observation
8. mid-upper arm circumference
9. urine
10. skin

11. x-ray films
12. height-weight
13. muscle mass
14. mid-upper arm muscle circumference

4.   The demand for _____ during childhood growth is relatively large, depending on the energy needs for _____ and the amount of _____. The main food source of energy for children is _____. It is also important as a _____ for their vital growth needs. The nine essential _____ are necessary in the child's diet to ensure proper tissue growth.

5.   A nutrient essential to life, second only to oxygen, is _____. Infants especially require attention to _____ balance because it comprises a greater percentage of their _____ and more of this amount is located_____; hence it is more easily _____.

1. carbohydrate
2. amino acids
3. basal metabolism
4. lost

5. water
6. physical activity
7. outside the cells
8. total body weight

9. kilocalories
10. protein-sparer

6.   Two main minerals needed during childhood are _____ for growth of bones and teeth, and _____ for formation of _____ to avoid anemia. Essential vitamins for growth include _____ for vision and epithelial tissue development, _____ for energy production and tissue building, _____ for cementing and strengthening developing tissue, _____ to aid the rapid bone development by absorbing and using the necessary _____, _____ to ensure blood clotting, and _____ to protect developing cell membrane structures. Excess amounts of _____ and _____ may have toxic effects.

1. B-complex vitamins
2. iron
3. vitamin K
4. vitamin E

5. vitamin C
6. hemoglobin
7. vitamin A
8. minerals

9. vitamin D
10. calcium

7.   Throughout the life cycle _____ and feeding practices not only serve to meet _____ for physical growth but also relate closely to personal _____ development during each stage of life. During infancy the core problem is the development of _____. Food becomes the baby's major vehicle of _____ with the environment and therefore of _____ of love and trust. _____ is the baby's first food, but it lacks _____; therefore, solid foods are needed by about 4-6 months of age to avoid _____ and to supply increased energy needs.

8.   After the first year, as the toddler begins to _____, his key psychosocial problem is the conflict between _____. He wants to do things for himself. Also, his physical growth rate has slowed. These two factors mean that the child needs _____ amounts of food for his size and will need to have some part in _____ his own food and feeding himself in his own way to meet the growing need for _____.

1. milk
2. iron
3. autonomy vs. shame
4. nutritional requirements
5. independence
6. selecting
7. trust vs. distrust
8. communication
9. walk
10. establishing relationships
11. food
12. anemia
13. smaller amounts
14. psychosocial

9.   The preschool child's psychosocial development centers on his struggle with the core problem of _____. His _____ is beginning to develop and _____ grows through imitation of _____ and their respective roles and habits. Mealtime and eating assume greater _____ aspects.

10.   For the school-age child, development of _____ capacities and increased _____ association with other children lead to the core psychosocial development problem of _____. The child eats more and more away from _____ with less dependence on _____ food habits. Often his meals are _____, consisting of snacks that are often _____.

1. conscience
2. motor and mental
3. home
4. sweets
5. initiative vs. guilt
6. irregular or skipped
7. sex identification
8. competitive
9. parents
10. industry vs. inferiority
11. family
12. social

11.   With the rapid body growth and _____ of adolescence, the key psychosocial development struggle is between _____. Physical growth_____, body composition changes, and _____ differences appear. The boy develops a greater _____, and the girl has a greater subcutaneous _____, which often leads her to great concern about _____. Teen-agers' tendency to follow _____ may result from pressure for group acceptance.

12.   It is evident throughout all these stage of growth and development that food habits do not develop only according to _____ needs. They are also directly related to _____ development and one's culture.

1. increases rapidly
2. sex
3. weight control
4. sex characteristic changes
5. physical growth
6. muscle mass
7. identity vs. role diffusion
8. food fads
9. psychosocial
10. fat deposit

122

Discussion Questions

1. Describe the degree of physical development of the premature infant at birth. How does this development relate to food choice and method of feeding?

2. Describe the process of lactation, both the preparation period during pregnancy and the initial breast-feeding of the infant.

3. Compare the commercial formulas for preterm and full-term infants. What differences do you see? Can you account for these differences?

4. What infant feeding practices may lead to infant and early childhood obesity, hence need reevaluation? What feeding practices would your suggest instead?

5. What food and feeding suggestions could you give to the parents of a preschool child to support his physical and psychosocial growth and development?

6. What nutrition problems is the teen-age girl likely to develop? Why?

Self-Test Questions

<u>True-False</u>
Circle the "T" if a statement is true and write a brief rationale for its accuracy. If it is false, circle the "F" and write the correct statement.

T F 1. A good way to avoid overweight infants and toddlers is to use nonfat milk in their diets.
T F 2. A variety of carbohydrate foods in the child's diet helps provide all the essential amino acids for growth.
T F 3. Iron, copper, and zinc work together to ensure the formation of hemoglobin and optimum growth.
T F 4. Calcium is needed in the child's diet for the formation of hemoglobin.
T F 5. Anemia may develop in an older infant fed too long on milk alone with no solid food additions.

T F 6. Hypervitaminosis C is possible during the growth period when an excess amount of the vitamin is given to infants.

T F 7. Colostrum, the premilk breast secretion, has limited nutritional value for the infant.

T F 8. Milk production and flow for breast-feeding is controlled by hormones from the pituitary gland.

T F 9. The rooting and sucking reflexes must be learned by the newborn infant before he can obtain milk from the breast.

T F 10. No particular food per se in the mother's diet influences milk production or disturbs the infant.

T F 11. The infant must develop sufficient muscular coordination of his tongue and swallowing reflex before he can manage to eat solid foods successfully.

T F 12. The toddler needs a quart of milk a day.

T F 13. Menstrual iron losses in the adolescent girl increase her risk of simple iron-deficiency anemia.

T F 14. Increased basal metabolism and thyroid activity during adolescence create a need for adequate iodine intake.

Multiple Choice

Circle the letter in front of the correct answer. Then check your answers by the test key (Appendix, p 264). Now compare all the possible answers for each item and write the following brief statements: (1) rationale for the correct answer and (2) why each one of the other responses is wrong.

1. Fat is needed in the child's diet to supply:
   - (1)   energy
   - (2)   fat-soluble vitamins
   - (3)   water-soluble vitamins
   - (4)   essential amino acids
   - (5)   essential fatty acids
   - a.   1, 2, and 5
   - b.   all of these
   - c.   3 and 5
   - d.   1 and 4

2. To meet growth demands, tissue protein can only by synthesized if:
   - (1)   the eight essential amino acids are supplied in the child's diet
   - (2)   these necessary amino acids are supplied in the correct proportion
   - (3)   all specific amino acids necessary for specific tissue protein are present in the body at the same time
   - (4)   the total dietary protein is sufficient in amount
   - a.   3 and 4
   - b.   1 and 2
   - c.   1 and 4
   - d.   all of these

124

3. Calcium is needed in a child's diet for:
   (1)   building bone tissue
   (2)   developing teeth
   (3)   proper blood coagulation
   (4)   aiding nerve-muscle function
   a.   all of these
   b.   1 and 2
   c.   3 and 4
   d.   1, 2, and 3
4. An iron deficiency in childhood is associated with the disease:
   a.   scurvy
   b.   rickets
   c.   anemia
   d.   pellagra
5. The growth and development of the school-age child are characterized by
   a.   a rapid increase in the physical growth, with increased food requirements
   b.   more rapid growth of girls in the latter part of the period
   c.   body changes associated with sexual maturity
   d.   increased dependence on parental standards or habits

Learning Activities
Individual Project: Nutrition for Growth

Select a child in one of the stages of growth from infancy through adolescence. Using the guidelines in your textbook, interview the mother and the child (depending on age) concerning the food and feeding practices used.

Analyze your findings using general guides in your textbook for each age group.

According to your findings, plan with the mother and the child (depending on age) a satisfying food plan that would help correct any deficiencies you may have identified and provide support for psychosocial development of the child.

Group-Teaching Project Infant Feeding

For a group of new mothers, plan and conduct a class on infant feeding. Discuss both breast-feeding and use of formulas. Have examples of different commercial formulas as examples. Include a cost comparison. Prepare your teaching plan to include the following parts:

1.   Breast-feeding and formulas
     a.   Teaching-learning objectives
     b.   Breast-feeding
     c.   Formulas
     d.   Results of class activity
     e.   Discussion, evaluation, and conclusions
2.   Solid food addition during the first year. (Use the same outline given above.)

<u>Individual or Group Project: Snack Foods for Growing Children</u>

Prepare a discussion for a group of parents of toddlers and preschool children. Develop snack ideas with recipes and suggestions for use. Demonstrate the preparation of a number of these snacks and have a taste-testing panel of the products with the parents. If children are present, have them taste and respond to the products.

Use the same general outline for your teaching-learning plan given previously.

<u>Situational Problem: Growth and Development of a Toddler</u>

Jimmy, a 2-year-old toddler, is active and "into everything." His constant desire to "do things for himself" is often a source of conflict with his mother. Often he lingers over his food without eating as much as his mother thinks he should.

1. What physical growth and development is Jimmy experiencing now?
2. What psychosocial problem is he facing? How is this affecting his behavior pattern?
3. What relation does his physical growth at this time and his psychosocial development (described above) have to:
   a. His nutrient requirements and reasons for them
   b. His food and feeding practices
   c. What suggestions would you make to his mother?

Current Nutritional Issues

Read carefully the *To Probe Further* box, "Food Habits of Adolescents" (*Essentials of Nutrition and Diet Therapy*, ed. 6 p 224; *Nutrition and Diet Therapy*, ed 7, p 385). Consider these inquiry questions:

1. What is your own observation of teenagers' eating habits? How would you evaluate these habits? Why?

2. Why do you think the number of fast-food chains has grown so rapidly? How would you evaluate these food items?

3. What unusual food choices or patterns have you observed among teenagers? Have you observed an increased use of alcohol and other drugs? How do you account for these trends and what dangers do they present?

4. How may some teenage girls suffer from the American obsession with thinness? What do you think may be some solutions to this problem?

126

Chapter 13
NUTRITION FOR ADULTS: EARLY, MIDDLE, AND LATER YEARS

Chapter Focus

Our growing numbers of older adults, many with burdens of chronic disease and insecure living situations, challenge our physical and psychosocial resources both as health care providers and as human beings. Nutritional support during these years becomes an increasingly important part of each person's care.

Summary-Review Quiz

Fill in the blanks below with the appropriate number and word(s) from the list following each section. Each numbered word or phrase is used; some may be used more than once. When you have completed all the sections, check your answers for each blank by the test key (Appendix, p 265). Correct any mistakes and then review the entire chapter summary.

1.   Aging is a very _____ process. It affects persons in _____ ways. It is an integral part of a person's _____ process and bears the accumulation of all _____ to that point.
2.   Psychosocial development during adulthood continues to influence _____ and behaviors, including _____. Young adults must resolve the core problem of _____ if they are to build meaningful _____, begin a family, or establish careers.
3.   In middle adulthood, with children out on their own, adults face the problem of _____. They must find some means of _____ of themselves and using their learning from life to help _____ find their way in turn. Finally, as an _____, each one must deal with his last personal life problem, that of _____. He may feel _____ or bitter, depending on his _____ and inner resources.

1. older adult
2. food behavior
3. generativity vs. self-absorption
4. personal relationships
5. integrity vs. despair
6. individual
7. younger persons
8. habits
9. intimacy vs. isolation
10. total life
11. life experiences
12. whole and complete
13. reaching out
14. different

4.   In American society, _____ value is given to elderly persons. This fact, together with the _____ of our culture, brings many _____ and _____ problems to older persons.

5.   From a biologic standpoint _____ changes occur with aging. Some of these changes may be sensory and affect _____ and amount of food eaten. Some may result from various types of _____ that also affect _____. These changes in food pattern affect _____. But since aging is an _____ process, these changes display a _____ of reactions. People simply get old at _____ and must be treated on an _____ basis.

1. appetite	6. different rates	11. nutritional status
2. psychologic	7. increasing complexity	12. socioeconomic
3. individual	8. wide variety	
4. food intake	9. stress	
5. less	10. physiologic	

6.   Among general nutritional requirements the need for _____ decreases in older age, but the need for _____ remains the same. It is wise for a good portion of the decreased fats in the adult diet to come from _____ plant fats rather than from _____ animal fats. On the other hand, at least _____ of the protein should be complete protein of _____ from _____ sources rather than incomplete forms from _____ sources. There is no need for _____ supplementation to these complete food sources. Generally for healthy adults there is no requirement for supplements of _____ and _____, except in specific cases of need as seen sometimes among the oldest-old group, so these _____ preparations are usually not necessary.

1. saturated	5. protein	9. half or more
2. plant	6. vitamins	10. minerals
3. high biologic value	7. unsaturated	11. kilocalories
4. expensive	8. amino acid	12. animal

7.   A basic clinical problem too often found in older adults in that of _____. Contributing factors include problems with _____ that make chewing difficult. Also there may be _____ problems that reduce appetite and food utilization. Other _____ problems such as loneliness, _____, or lack of _____ or transportation to obtain food may create more difficulty. Additional clinical problems may include _____ problems such as heart disease or _____, which may cause difficulties with _____ needs.

8.   Solutions to these problems vary with the _____ situation. In any situation the guiding principle is that of maintaining the _____ of each person as much as possible and using a variety of _____ to provide needed services or assistance.

1. personal	5. malnutrition	9. chronic disease
2. modified diet	6. diabetes mellitus	10. inadequate housing
3. money	7. community resources	11. individual
4. personal integrity	8. teeth or dentures	12. gastrointestinal

Discussion Questions

1.   What social and economic problems may adults in each age group—early, middle, and later years—face in American society?

2.   What possible solutions to these problems can you suggest?

3.   Why do you think cases of actual malnutrition are often discovered among older adults?

4.   Describe the Nutrition Screening Initiative program and its identified risk factors as warning signs of malnutrition in older adults. Why do you think older adults may be at special risk of malnutrition? Can you describe such an elderly person you may know from your own experience? What available assistance programs for older Americans may be helpful to such persons? What type of help does each program provide?

5.   How does nutrition relate to the major chronic diseases of adult life? Give some examples. Why do you think many physicians are relaxing the use of "medically indicated" diets for elderly persons and focusing more on well-balanced regular diets for good nutrition?

Self-Test Questions

True-False

Circle the "T" if a statement is true and write a brief rationale for its accuracy. If it is false, circle the "F" and write the correct statement.

T F 1. The needs and problems of the young-old (ages 60 to 75 years) adult may be quite different from those of the old-old (over 75 years) adult.

T F 2. Old persons in American society are generally given much value and made to feel needed and productive.

T F 3. In American health care much progress has been made in the control of chronic disease in old age and related medical and social care practices in meeting the needs of the aged.

T F 4. Beginning about the age of 30, a gradual increase occurs in the performance capacity of most organ systems throughout adulthood.

T F 5. The average adult requires about 1800 kilocalories daily to meet his energy demands.

T F 6. The simplest basis for judging adequacy of caloric intake is the maintenance of normal weight.

T F 7. The protein requirement increases with age.

T F 8. Most elderly persons require additional supplements of vitamins and minerals.

T F 9. Older persons are frequent victims of food faddists' claims.

Multiple Choice

Circle the letter in front of the correct answer. Then check your answers by the test key (Appendix, p 266). Now compare all the possible answers for each item and write the following brief statements: (1) rationale for the correct answer and (2) why each one of the other responses is wrong.

1. American population changes include:
    (1)   an increasing number of persons 65 years of age
    (2)   a general increase in total population, although the current rate has slowed somewhat
    (3)   a decreasing number of persons over 65 years of age
    (4)   an overall decline in our total population
    a.   1 and 2
    b.   3 and 4
    c.   1 and 4
    d.   2 and 3

2. Basic needs of older persons include:
   - (1) economic security
   - (2) a sense of personal self-worth and productivity
   - (3) suitable and comfortable housing
   - (4) positive social relationships and some kind of constructive leisure-time activities
   - (5) some satisfying spiritual values and personal goals
   - a. 1, 2, and 3
   - b. 1, 3, and 4
   - c. 2, 4, and 5
   - d. all of these

3. The basic biologic changes in older adults include:
   - a. an increase in number of cells
   - b. a decreasing sense of self-worth
   - c. an increased basal metabolic rate
   - d. a gradual loss of functioning cells and reduced cell metabolism

4. Which of the following responses give examples of physiologic changes in aging?
   - (1) after a stress load of sugar, such as in a glucose tolerance test, the blood sugar returns to normal more rapidly
   - (2) after exercise the pulse rate and respiration take longer to return normal
   - (3) a gradual increase in the body's reserve capacity
   - (4) there may be decreased gastrointestinal function
   - a. 2 and 4
   - b. 1 and 3
   - c. 1 and 2
   - d. 3 and 4

5. Protein needs in adulthood are influenced by:
   - (1) the biologic value of the dietary protein being used
   - (2) adequacy of the diet's energy value (kcalories)
   - (3) the person's state of health
   - (4) the nature of the dietary fats being used—the saturated to unsaturated ratio
   - a. 1, 2, and 3
   - b. 1, 3, and 4
   - c. 3, 4, and 5
   - d. all of these

6. Personal factors contributing to nutritional problems in older persons include:
   - (1) limited financial resources
   - (2) lack of transportation to a food market
   - (3) inadequate housing with poor cooking and food storage facilities
   - (4) some degree of physical disability or social isolation
   - a. 1, 2, and 3
   - b. all of these
   - c. 2, 3, and 4
   - d. 1, 3, and 4

7. Which of the following attitudes and actions would be most helpful in assisting an elderly person to find solutions to health problems?
   (1)   analyzing the individual living situation and food habits carefully
   (2)   reinforcing good habits, leaving harmless ones alone, and making suggestions for those things needing change within the practical reality of individual living situations
   (3)   encouraging as much variety as possible in foods and seasonings
   (4)   exploring and using any available community resources for assistance
   a.   1 and 4
   b.   2 and 3
   c.   3 and 4
   d.   all of these

Learning Activities

Individual or Small-Group (Two or Three Persons) Project: Nutritional Analysis of an Older Adult's Diet

Select an elderly person and plan, if possible, a home visit. In the home, interview this person and make observations concerning food use and habits. For example, go with the person into the kitchen and evidence interest in facilities for food preparation and storage. Note the food products on shelves or otherwise available for use.

Analyze your findings in terms of three basic nutrients—protein, vitamin C, and iron—as well as energy (kcalories) intake. Also note the nature of the carbohydrates (complex, simple, fiber) and fats (animal or plant sources) being used.

Plan with the person a suitable diet with suggestions to accommodate: (1) nutritional needs, (2) personal desires, (3) variety in foods and seasonings, and (4) the practical living situation.

Accompany the person to a nearby market, if possible, to help make suggestions concerning wise buying of food products. Return to the home and help prepare a demonstration meal or snacks, showing nutrition values. Follow up with a later visit to evaluate the results of your diet counseling.

Individual Project: Health Food Store Survey

Visit a nearby community health food store. Note any products that seem particularly marketed for elderly persons. Study the labels on food items and the nature of the advertising.

Make a similar visit to a drugstore and locate any vitamin or mineral preparations that may be labeled *geriatric*. Read the label and any advertising claims.

Evaluate your findings in terms of your knowledge at this point of nutritional needs for elderly persons.

Individual or Small Group Project: Old-age Assistance Programs

Visit your community welfare department and public health department to interview a social worker or a public health nutritionist concerning the following old-age assistance programs in operation in your community: (1) Social Security, (2) Medicare, (3) food stamps, and (4) community feeding programs.

Evaluate each of these programs in terms of adequacy in meeting the needs of elderly persons in your community. Discuss in your interview how each of the programs works, what the eligibility requirements are, and how many persons are being reached by each of the programs. Prepare an oral report of your finding for your class.

Individual or Group Project: Community Senior Citizen's Center

Arrange an informal meeting or social gathering at your local senior citizen's center for a group of your class members. Discuss with them informally the activities at the center.

Later, in your class discussion of your experiences, evaluate the senior citizen's program that you discovered at the center in terms of the member's participation and benefits.

If the group desires, plan a demonstration of nutritious tasteful food snacks with suggestions for economical food buying. Use the following items for planning your food demonstration: (1) objectives, (2) materials needed, (3) procedure, (4) results, and (5) discussions and conclusions. Make an oral or written report to your class of the results of your experience.

Situational Problem: Nutritional Needs of an Elderly Woman

Mrs. Baker is a 78-year-old widow, living alone in a three-bedroom house in a large city. A fall 1 year ago resulted in a broken hip, and she is now dependent on a walker for limited mobility. Her husband died suddenly 6 months ago, and almost all her friends are deceased or disabled. Her only daughter lives in a distant city and apparently does not care to bear the burden of responsibility for her mother.

Mrs. Baker's only income is a monthly Social Security check for $160. Her monthly property taxes, insurance, and utilities are $130.

A recent medical examination revealed that Mrs. Baker is severely anemic and that she has lost 20 pounds in the past 3 months. Her current weight is 82 pounds, and she is 5 feet 4 inches tall. She states that she has not been hungry and her daily diet is now quite repetitious: bouillon, a little cottage cheese and canned fruit, saltines, and hot tea. She lacks energy, rarely leaves the house, and appears emaciated and generally distraught.

1. What core psychosocial problem confronts Mrs. Baker and how might it have influenced her eating habits?

2. What nutritional improvements could she make in her diet (include food suggestions), and how are they related to her physical needs at this stage of her life?

3.   What practical suggestions do you have for assisting Mrs. Baker in coping with her physical and social environment? For example, consider use of personal and community resources, income, food, and companionship. How do you think these suggestions will benefit her nutritional and overall health status?

Current Nutrition Issues

Read carefully the *Issues and Answers* article, "Can We Eat to Live Forever?" (*Essentials of Nutrition and Diet Therapy*, ed 6, p 267; *Nutrition and Diet Therapy*, ed 7, p 410). Consider these inquiry questions:

1. What problems do you see that may have been caused by American medicine's advance in lengthening our lifespan?

2. Why is defining an optimal diet for elderly persons such a difficult task?

3. Why do you think many older adults take vitamin-mineral supplements, even in megadoses? How would you evaluate these practices?

4. What problems do some elderly persons face that may contribute to their poor nutrition? Can you suggest some solutions to these problems?

Chapter 14
NUTRITION AND PHYSICAL FITNESS

Chapter Focus

Both nutrition and physical exercise relate to energy balance. One provides the fuel input and metabolic control agents. The other, along with basal metabolic work, accounts for energy output. Thus these two factors, nutrition and physical activity, are essential to physical fitness. They are closely interrelated not only in health maintenance but also in disease prevention and control.

Summary-Review Quiz

Fill in the blanks below with the appropriate number and word(s) from the list following each section. Each numbered word or phrase is used; some may be used more than once. When you have completed all the sections, check your answers for each blank by the test key (Appendix, p 266). Correct any mistakes and then review the entire chapter summary.

1.   The term _____ refers to the body's ability to do work, both _____ activity and _____ activity. This _____ is constantly being _____ and cycled in the body and its environment to do a variety of _____.

2.   This working power may be stored as _____ or in an active use as _____. Our food supplies _____, which together with _____ and _____ provide _____ demands for body needs.

1. transformed	5. potential energy	9. energy
2. kinetic energy	6. metabolic	10. body work
3. physical	7. oxygen	
4. water	8. substrate fuels	

3.   Finely coordinated _____ and _____ make up our muscle structures. The total _____ makes possible all of our _____ activity.

4.   The parallel rows of contractile proteins, _____ and _____, in the _____ slide together to _____ then pull apart to _____, as regular _____ takes place. Muscle _____ occurs due to (1) depletion of the fuel supply of _____ or (2) accumulation of _____ from muscle action.

1. skeletal muscle mass
2. lactic acid
3. relax
4. myosin

5. muscle glycogen
6. specialized cells
7. muscle action
8. physical

9. contract
10. muscle fibers
11. fatigue
12. actin

5.   The main high-energy compound of body cells is _____. It is rightly called the _____ of the cell. Fuel for immediate energy needs is supplied by _____ and its backup compound _____.

6.   Fuel for _____ energy needs is supplied by _____. But this amount is _____ and lasts a _____ time. Fuel for long-term energy needs is supplied by large amounts of _____, mainly from _____ metabolism of _____ and _____.

1. muscle glycogen
2. fatty acids
3. energy currency
4. short-term

5. glucose
6. creatine phosphate (CP)
7. short
8. oxygen-dependent

9. ATP
10. small

7.   Increased sweating during exercise causes _____. A deficiency of _____ can lead to the serious complication of _____. Continued exercise depletes _____ as the body burns _____ and _____ to provide energy. Prolonged exercise reduces these _____ to dangerous levels bringing _____ and eventual _____.

8.   The most _____ to a person's exercise level is the ability to deliver _____ to tissues. This ability depends on fitness of the _____ and _____ systems. This _____ depends on degree of (1) _____ and (2) _____, the relative amounts of body fat and _____. Persons with a higher percentage of _____ have a greater _____. Exercise helps to lower _____ and increase _____, and hence increases _____.

1. nutrients
2. fuels
3. physical fitness
4. lean body mass
5. exhaustion
6. water

7. oxygen
8. cardiovascular
9. blood glucose
10. muscle fatigue
11. pulmonary
12. limiting factor

13. body fat
14. water loss
15. body composition
16. muscle glycogen
17. aerobic capacity
18. dehydration

9.   Our diet supplies the necessary _____ for energy needs. We require _____ and _____ as basic _____ but use _____ amounts of _____ during exercise. Diets high in _____ lead to (1) increased production and excretion of urea which contributes to serious _____ and (2) increased excretion and loss of _____.

10. Fat as a _____ is not drawn directly from the _____ but from _____. Thus we do not need to eat more fat than just our _____ to burn fat as _____. We do need some fat in the _____, however, as a source of the _____ fatty acid, _____, but the total fat amount should not exceed _____ of the total daily kcalorie intake.

1. fuel	6. essential	11. linoleic acid
2. dehydration	7. protein	12. fuel substrate
3. body fat stores	8. calcium	13. diet
4. 24% to 30%	9. dietary needs	14. fat
5. carbohydrate	10. insignificant	

11. The major _____ for energy needs is _____. It should contribute about _____ of the daily caloric intake. The preferred form is _____ to provide a more sustained source of the immediate fuels _____ and _____. Less efficient are the _____, because they (1) do not maintain _____ stores as well and (2) provoke a sharper _____ response, which together with the _____ increases the risk of _____.

12. Vitamins and minerals cannot be used as _____ but they are essential in _____ as _____ factors. Exercise raises the body's need for _____ and regulates _____ to meet these needs.

1. blood glucose	6. carbohydrate	11. fuel substrate
2. 55%	7. energy production	12. insulin
3. exercise	8. hypoglycemia	13. kcalories
4. simple sugars	9. coenzyme	14. complex carbohydrate
5. appetite	10. muscle glycogen	

Discussion Questions

1. Why do you think athletes and coaches are so susceptible to myths and magic claims about foods and supplements?

2. What is the theory behind the glycogen-loading practice of athletes? Why does this practice carry some dangers from too frequent use?

3. What is the ideal pregame meal? Why?

137

4. Why does the endurance athlete have to pay special attention to adequate water supply? What problems may arise? How may they be prevented?

5. Would you recommend a "sports drink" (such as Gatorade) with added electrolytes and glucose to an athlete for rehydration? Support your answer.

Self-Test Questions

<u>True-False</u>
    Circle the "T" if a statement is true and write a brief rationale for its accuracy. If it is false, circle the "F" and write the correct statement.

T F 1. Water containing electrolytes and sugar is the best way to replace these substances lost during typical sports and exercise periods.
T F 2. Cold water is absorbed more quickly from the stomach.
T F 3. Drinking water immediately before or during an athletic event causes cramps.
T F 4. Athletes need protein for extra energy.
T F 5. Vitamins and minerals are burned up for energy in workouts and training sessions.
T F 6. Protein and fat do not contribute to glycogen stores
T F 7. Sweating is our main mechanism for dissipating body heat.
T F 8. Aerobic exercise is of limited benefit in control of heart disease or diabetes.
T F 9. To build aerobic exercise, the exercise level must raise the pulse to within 70% of maximum heart rate.
T F 10. Walking can be an excellent form of aerobic exercise.

<u>Multiple Choice</u>
    Circle the letter in front of the correct answer. Then check your answers by the test key (Appendix, p 267). Now compare all the possible answers for each item and write the following brief statements: (1) rationale for the correct answer and (2) why each one of the other responses is wrong.

1. Which of the following general activities is most likely to provide aerobic exercise?
    a.   golf
    b.   swimming
    c.   tennis
    d.   baseball

2. To develop aerobic capacity the exercise should:
    a.   raise the pulse to 50% of maximal heart rate
    b.   be maintained for intermittent periods of 10 minutes each
    c.   be practiced consistently every day
    d.   be practiced three to five times a week at appropriate pulse rate for sustained periods of time
3. Characteristics of a healthful exercise program include:
    a.   enjoyable activity
    b.   moderation
    c.   regularity
    d.   all of these
4. The primary benefit of exercise in diabetes control is:
    a.   control of hypoglycemia in IDDM
    b.   increased number of insulin receptor sites in NIDDM
    c.   decreased weight in IDDM
    d.   better balance with insulin dosage in NIDDM
5. Exercise is beneficial in weight management because it:
    (1)   helps regulate appetite
    (2)   decreases the BMR
    (3)   reduces stress-related eating
    (4)   increases the "set-point" level for fat deposit
    a.   1 and 3
    b.   2 and 4
    c.   1 and 4
    d.   2 and 3
6. Which of the following effects does exercise have on bone disease?
    (1)   reduces bone weakness
    (2)   increases bone mineralization
    (3)   increases withdrawal of bone calcium
    (4)   decreases muscle tension on bones
    a.   1 and 4
    b.   2 and 3
    c.   1 and 2
    d.   3 and 4
7. Which of these meals would be the best choice as a pregame meal for athletes?
    a.   large grilled steak, fried potatoes, ice cream
    b.   fried fish, tossed salad, fresh fruit
    c.   spaghetti with tomato sauce, French bread, fruit
    d.   hamburger, french fries, cola

8. The best nutrient percentages of total kilocalories in a diet for support of physical activity are:
   a.   15% protein, 30% fat, 55% carbohydrate
   b.   20% protein, 50% fat, 30% carbohydrate
   c.   30% protein, 10% fat, 60% carbohydrate
   d.   40% protein, 20% fat, 40% carbohydrate

Learning Activities

Individual or Small Group Project: Nutritional Analysis of Athletes' Diets

Select two athletes in your school or community, one male and one female, and interview them about their food habits and attitudes, use of supplements, pregame meals, any nutrition advice from coaches, and any other food-related practices.

Analyze your findings in terms of total energy value of diet (kilocalories and relative percentages of total kilocalories supplied by protein, fat, and carbohydrate.

Compare the two athlete's diets, nutrition practices, and beliefs.

Present your findings to the class.

Follow-up your initial interview with any dietary counseling indicated, if it is appropriate.

Group Project: Discussion Group for Athletes

Plan with a school or community organization athletic director to hold an informal discussion group with team members to present nutritional information for athletes and answer their questions about food and nutrient practices or beliefs.

Provide a display of sound nutrition resources and reference lists for sources of helpful materials.

Group Project: Fitness Center

Visit a variety of fitness centers in your community as potential customers. Gather information and reference materials about the center's program: services offered, costs involved, staff resources, and diet recommendations or sale of any nutrients in relation to their program.

Compare and evaluate these programs in a follow-up class discussion.

Current Nutritional Issues

Read carefully the *Issues and Answers* article, "The Winning Edge—or Over the Edge?" (*Essentials of Nutrition and Diet Therapy*, ed 6, p 283; *Nutrition and Diet Therapy*, ed 7, p 430). Consider these inquiry questions:

1. Why do some athletes try to maintain as low a percentage of body fat as possible? What is the danger in this practice?

2. Why would young athletes or female athletes be especially at risk form this low body fat attempt?

3. Why do you think most compulsive runners are men?

4. How is the self-concept associated with these problems? What solutions can you suggest?

Chapter 15
NUTRITION AND STRESS MANAGEMENT

Chapter Focus

Rapidly changing and fast-paced life in technologic societies such as America's produces stressful pressures and problems for many people. These stresses bring immediate physiologic responses and long-term psychosocial effects, as well as community environmental concerns, both of which affect our nutritional needs and health. This stress in modern life plays an increasing risk-factor role in our so-called diseases of civilization—heart disease, cancer, diabetes, and hypertension.

Summary-Review Quiz

Fill in the blanks below with the appropriate number and word(s) from the list following each section. Each numbered word or phrase is used; some may be used more than once. When you have completed all the sections, check your answers for each blank by the test key (Appendix, p 268). Correct any mistakes and then review the entire chapter summary.

1. Early classic research of _____, strongly reinforced by later studies, shows the close relation of _____ to health maintenance and disease. Varying effects of _____ on different individuals depend on _____, such as personal genetics, _____, or on external influences such as _____ and _____ or other _____. Thus, _____ and management has become a vital consideration in _____ and _____.
2. Normal _____ is a part of life's constant change and balance. Automatic _____ maintain the body's dynamic balance or _____.
3. But prolonged _____ contributes to depletion of human resources and _____. Four basic areas of human need can relate to this state: (1) _____, (2) _____, (3) _____, and (4) _____.

1. alcohol
2. health promotion
3. physiologic stress
4. conditioning factors
5. life-cycle growth and development
6. stress assessment
7. human self-fulfillment needs
8. illness
9. Selye
10. stress-coping balance

11. drug abuse
12. age or sex
13. uncontrolled stress
14. health-disease status
15. physiologic responses
16. disease treatment
17. poor diet
18. homeostasis
19. stress

4. The work of _____ has identified three distinct stages of the human physiologic _____, which together have been called the body's _____.

5. In the first stage, the brain's _____ mobilizes the body's forces for immediate _____. This alarm is carried from the brain by its chemical messengers, the _____. These initial agents operate on the brain's _____ to trigger in turn still other chemical _____ and _____, which adapt and change the body's _____, releasing its _____ to combat the perceived danger.

1. neurotransmitters	5. hormones	9. protective action
2. nutrient reserves	6. initial alarm reaction	10. general adaptive syndrome
3. response to stress	7. hypothalamus	
4. normal physiology	8. Selye	

6. In the second stage, marked _____ follow the initial alarm reaction. Here _____ reserves are _____ to strengthen the body's _____. Normal _____ cuts off continued initial _____ for a return to normal levels. The necessary restoring of body _____ require positive _____ and general personal _____.

7. In the third stage, _____ resources may reach the point of _____. If this condition is not relieved, _____ will ultimately occur. The body's _____ becomes depressed and thus is more vulnerable to _____.

8. This this third stage, special white cells called _____ diminish in number and can no longer adequately defend the body against invading _____. This failing _____ can result from individual _____ such as _____ and _____.

1. hormonal feedback	7. lymphocytes	13. stress tolerance
2. adjusted and rebuilt	8. tissue reserves	14. malnutrition
3. coping powers	9. poor health	15. hormonal output
4. death	10. exhaustion	16. disease-producing antigens
5. energy	11. nutritional support	17. resistance and adaptation
6. conditioning factors	12. disease	18. stress-coping
		19. immune function

9. Each life cycle stage of growth and development carries both _____ and _____ nutrition-related stress. During pregnancy normal _____ to support new life brings added stress. Other stress factors include _____ and socioeconomic concerns to meet changing personal roles as _____.

10. Other stress factors contribute to high-risk pregnancy. Some may exist before the pregnancy: (1) _____ extremes, (2) _____ pregnancies, or (3) poor _____. Added stress factors may come from social problems such as _____ and a resulting _____, or from harmful personal habits such as use of _____, _____, or _____.

11. Still further stress may come from pregnancy complications such as _____ or _____, or from preexisting maternal disease such as _____ or _____. These clinical conditions require special _____.

1. age
2. drug abuse
3. lack of prenatal care
4. maternal phenylketonuria (MPKU)
5. parents
6. alcohol
7. obstetrical history
8. insulin-dependent diabetes mellitus (IDDM)
9. psychosocial
10. nutritional support
11. smoking
12. physiologic adaptation
13. physiologic
14. pregnancy-induced hypertension (PIH)
15. frequent
16. anemia
17. poverty

12. After the stress of birth, _____ face the stress of the external world and require both _____ and _____ of loving care and appropriate feeding.
13. High-risk infants may suffer the effects of _____ from either _____ or some some sort of _____. Other high-risk infants may have _____. Still others suffer general _____, sometimes due to defective _____ interaction. All of these infants require careful _____ as a basis for planning special nutritional care.

1. low birth weight
2. birth defects
3. prematurity
4. psychosocial nurturing
5. nutritional and social assessment
6. failure to thrive
7. newborns
8. intrauterine growth retardation (IUGR)
9. physiologic nourishment
10. mother-infant

14. During childhood, physical growth places _____ stress demands on young bodies and _____ adds personal stress. Food and mealtimes become important as a means of _____.
15. High-risk children suffer added _____ stress. Such stress may come from: (1) _____, (2) _____, or (3) _____.
16. Rapid adolescent growth and sexual maturation bring _____ and great stress to teenagers from related _____. Added health risks may come from: (1) _____, (2) _____, (3) _____, (4) _____, or (5) _____.

1. body changes
2. growth failure
3. teenage pregnancies
4. drug abuse
5. chronic genetic disease
6. physiologic and psychosocial
7. athletic pressures
8. socialization
9. eating disorders
10. psychosocial development
11. alcohol
12. emotional and social tensions
13. developmental disability
14. metabolic

Discussion Questions

1. Why does growth and development during childhood and adolescence often bring stress to many children? How do the normal stages of psychosocial development relate to these stresses? Describe these stages and the basic psychosocial developmental task at each stage and related problems.

2. What environmental changes have you observed in your community? In other communities? How have these increased environmental stress factors brought health risks?

3. Physical exercise contributes to health. But can heavy or compulsive exercise become a high-stress risk factor? How? Give some examples.

4. Identify stress factors in the workplace that can contribute to injury, illness, or disease. Describe any such situations you may have experienced or know about. How do you think such stress-related problems could be solved?

5. Describe the high-risk problems of physical and mental stress due to poverty and hunger that you have observed in your community. Why do you think these problems exist in a wealthy developed country? What solutions can you propose?

6. How can stress contribute to mental health problems? In what ways may these problems contribute to nutritional problems?

Self-Test Questions

True-False

Circle the "T" if a statement is true and write a brief rationale for its accuracy. If it is false, circle the "F" and write the correct statement.

T F 1. Specific stress factors usually cause the same stress reaction in most persons.

T F 2. Our "fight or flight" response to stress works as well to protect us today as it did in the primitive times of its development.

T F 3. Normal physiologic stress is a vital part of human interaction with a changing environment.

T F 4. Severe prolonged stress contributes to exhaustion of human resources and eventual illness.

T F 5. Objective data such as pain, tolerances, feelings about health status and problems provide clearly measured information on which to plan general care.

T F 6. In physiologic stress a number of automatic body responses maintain homeostasis.

T F 7. In psychosocial stress these automatic physiologic coping responses also act to maintain a healthful balance.

T F 8. Persons usually perceive a given stress in the same way and respond to it in like manner.

T F 9. Emotional tension from multiple causes is the most common agent of human stress.

T F 10. The effect of any life stressor depends on its nature, duration, and the strength of personal coping resources.

Multiple Choice

Circle the letter in front of the correct answer. Then check your answers by the test key (Appendix, p 269). Now compare all the possible answers for each item and write the following brief statements: (1) rationale for the correct answer, and (2) why each one of the other responses is wrong.

1. Neurotransmitters of stress signals from the brain act in which of the following ways to warn the body of danger?
   a. Go immediately to various body tissues, causing them to adapt their normal physiologic functions to meet the danger.
   b. Travel along a single prescribed route to speed the body's reaction rate.
   c. Go immediately from brain cortex to the hypothalamus for automatic redirection through two separate neuroendocrine tracks to meet needs.
   d. Travel to body tissues through the central nervous system to reach all parts of the body.

2. Chemical agents of the body's combined neuroendocrine system immediately responding to stress include which of the following substances?
   (1) Hormones
   (2) Special hormone-releasing factor
   (3) Catecholamines
   (4) Stored tissue fuels
   a. 1, 2, and 3
   b. 1, 3, and 4
   c. 1, 2, and 4
   d. 2, 3, and 4

3. Protective physiologic responses to the body's initial alarm reaction to stress include which of the following effects?
   (1) Increases pulse and respiration
   (2) Mobilizes emergency tissue fuels for energy
   (3) Increases blood pressure
   (4) Guards body water
   (5) Makes fuel available to muscles and brain
   a. 1, 3, and 5
   b. 2, 4, and 5
   c. 3, 4, and 5
   d. all of these

4. In the follow-up stress response stage of resistance and adaptation, which of the following reactions occur?
   (1) A hormonal feedback mechanism cuts off initial hormone output.
   (2) Blood levels of the initial alarm-responding neuroendocrine agents remain elevated for continued protection.
   (3) Depleted body tissue reserves are rebuilt.
   (4) Lost body weight is regained.
   a. 1, 2, and 4
   b. 2, 3, and 4
   c. 1, 3, and 4
   d. 1, 2, and 3

5. In the final stress-response stage of exhaustion of stress-coping resources, which of the following effects occur?
   (1) The body's immune system weakens.
   (2) The numbers of special white cells, the T and B cell lymphocytes the fight disease, diminish.
   (3) Disease follows if individual conditioning factors, such as poor health and nutrition, are present.
   (4) Death follows if resources are not restored.
   a. 1 and 2
   b. 2 and 3
   c. 3 and 4
   d. all of these

Learning Activities

Group Project: Community Nutritional Support Programs

In partners or small groups, investigate various community programs that are helping to meet the needs of persons, especially families with young children, that are without incomes or homes, or are living in depressed conditions of poverty. Contact the director or nutritionist, or other staff person, and make an appointment to learn about their program. Make out ahead a list of inquiry questions to structure your interview. Include a discussion of needs, extent of this problem in the community, how the program is trying to meet these needs, what problems they are encountering, and possible solutions that may be available. How may you make any contributions of time, goods, or services—individually or as a class project?

Individual Project: Developing a Personal Stress Management Plan

Read carefully the chapter section on "High-Risk Stress Management." Follow the process involved of self-assessment and develop a personal stress management plan. Include possible social approaches and support groups, personal lifestyle approach involving physical activities, relaxation exercises or activities, and diet assessment including nutritional balance, relation of food and mood, food pattern and pace, socioeconomic needs, or any hypermetabolic needs that may exist.

After assessment and planning for your own stress-reduction needs, consider any person you know who is experiencing particular stress and help them follow the same approach of assessing their own situation. Then support their efforts in making a similar personal plan, using nourishing diet, physical exercise, and relaxation exercises to better manage stress in their lives.

Keep a journal of these experiences and plans, if even for a brief period, as a means of measuring progress toward personal goals, gaining insights about self, and assessing movement toward health and nutrition goals involved.

Current Nutrition Issues

Read carefully the *Issues and Answers* article, "Social Isolation and Health" (*Essentials of Nutrition and Diet Therapy*, ed 6, p 302; *Nutrition and Diet Therapy*, ed 7, p 452). Consider these inquiry questions:

1.   Why does social isolation contribute to stress-related health risks?

2.   How does such social isolation relate to nutrition problems?

3.   What changes in our society are adding to this problem of isolation? How are social contacts and relationships an important part of health? What clinical evidence supports this association?

4.   How does this pattern relate to our major health problems?

5.   Describe ways in which social relationships affect health and the quality of our lives. How do the factors of age, race, sex, and socioeconomic status affect social isolation? What are the implications for community health care?

Chapter 16
NUTRITIONAL ASSESSMENT AND THERAPY IN PATIENT CARE

Chapter Focus

Sound nutritional therapy during hospitalization, directed by the clinical nutritionist and physician on the health care team, is essential support to medical treatment and to the patient's personal well-being. To be realistic, this nutritional care must be *person-centered*, based on comprehensive assessment data.

Summary-Review Quiz

Fill in the blanks below with the appropriate number and word(s) from the list following each section. Each numbered word or phrase is used; some may be used more than once. When you have completed all the sections, check your answers for each blank by the test key (Appendix, p 269). Correct any mistakes and then review the entire chapter summary.

1.   Diet therapy is based on _____ needs. Thus a _____ diet is modified from the _____ diet only insofar as is necessary to meet a specific _____ requirement. The needs of hospitalized persons are influenced by three factors: (1) the patient's _____, (2) the limitations and resources of the _____, and (3) the various functions and relationships of the _____.

2.   A patient's needs arise from: (1) physical causes based on the _____ or health problem; (2) psychologic causes based on _____ concerning the illness and hospitalization and _____ with these anxieties; (3) from social causes based on _____ situation; or (4) additional stress based on the _____ of _____ and _____.

1. disease
2. hospital staff
3. frustrations and fears
4. normal nutritional
5. modern medicine
6. family or business
7. illness
8. hospital setting
9. therapeutic
10. high costs
11. personal needs and goals
12. hospital care
13. inability to cope
14. normal

3.   Nutritional care is always planned on the individual patient's _____. The nutritional diagnosis and _____ is directed by the patient's _____ and _____. Sources of information to determine needs are (1) the _____ and family; (2) the _____; and (3) the _____ and other _____ helping to provide the patient care and support services. Nutritional needs of patients may be found in the influences of _____ recorded or reviewed in histories, _____ at the time of hospitalization, and _____ for continuing care after

discharge.

4.   The clinical nutritionist uses several basic types of assessment means: (1) _____ measures; (2) _____ and other test results; (3) _____ observations and _____ examination; (4)_____ evaluations; (5) careful _____ history; (6) all _____ and any food- or nutrient-drug _____; and (7) full _____ history.

1. patient's medical chart
2. clinical
3. present needs
4. physician
5. personal-family-social
6. hospital staff
7. biochemical
8. dietary
9. plan of care
10. interactions
11. past experiences
12. clinical nutritionist
13. anthropometric
14. drug therapy
15. physical
16. health needs
17. medical
18. health care team
19. future needs
20. patient

5.   Based on _____ of the full _____, a list of _____ is identified and related plan of care is developed around these personal needs and _____.   Follow-up _____ and _____ of results allows for change in care as needed.

6.   The members of the _____ working with the patient contribute to the care plan.   It needs to be _____ and modified according to _____. Involvement of the _____ in planning care is essential.

1. problems
2. recording
3. patient
4. health care team
5. assessment database
6. continued observations
7. analysis
8. evaluation
9. flexible
10. goals

7.   A therapeutic diet may be modified in: (1) one or more of the basic _____; (2) in total _____ value as expressed in _____; or (3) in _____ or seasoning.

8.   Information needed to plan a valid therapeutic diet includes: (1) knowledge of the _____ and its effects on the normal body functions; (2) how the _____ of the diet need to be modified; (3) how daily _____ and preparation can meet these diet _____; and (4) how this diet can be adapted to the _____. Alternative modes of feeding by gastrointestinal _____ or by _____ may have to be used.

9.   Routine hospital diets vary mainly in _____, including the simplest form-- a _____ diet, which may be full or clear, depending on the use of milk; a _____ diet which would include mainly cooked foods and have bland seasonings; and a _____ diet, which would include all foods for a normal well balanced diet.

1. disease
2. patient's life situation
3. modifications
4. nutrients
5. vein

6. texture
7. regular
8. nutritional components
9. soft
10. energy

11. liquid
12. food choices
13. tube
14. kcalories

10.   To meet the basic overall objective in serving food to patients, two guiding principles apply: (1) all diets are _____, whether they are regular _____ or special _____, and thus should provide the necessary base for _____ and health and (2) no food can accomplish these health objectives unless it is served to the patient and the patient _____ it. Therefore the _____ needs of the patient must also be met and assistance and _____ provided whenever necessary. Often the involvement of the patient's _____ is helpful.

11.   Since continuing of good food habits based on a knowledge of individual dietary needs is important to the patient's health, _____ opportunities should be sought. These teaching opportunities may include simple _____ concerning food and nutritional values and needs; use of the hospital's selective _____ and the _____ served, for guiding food choices and values; discussion with the patient's _____, especially the one who will be responsible for _____ after the patient is discharged; and exploration of _____ resources available to provide assistance.

1. personal
2. nutrition education
3. tray food
4. special therapeutic diets
5. food preparation

6. menu
7. therapy
8. family
9. support
10. hospital and community

11. hospital diets
12. healing
13. planned conversation
14. accepts and eats

Discussion Questions

1.   What factors influence the hospitalized patient's acceptance or rejection of his food? Compare the needs of an adult patient with those of a child.

2.   Name some specific observations you could make concerning a patient's relation to the food served him in the hospital. How could you use these observations to help you in planning this patient's nutritional therapy and education?

3. Suggest some ways that you could help a child in the pediatric ward accept and enjoy his food. What needs of the child would this food acceptance and enjoyment achieve?

4. Suggest some ways that you could help a patient learn about his nutritional needs.

5. A significant amount of frank malnutrition has been observed in hospitalized patients. What factors do you think may contribute to this situation? What could be done to prevent it?

Self-Test Questions

<u>True-False</u>
    Circle the "T" if a statement is true and write a brief rationale for its accuracy. If it is false, circle the "F" and write the correct statement.

T F   1. The basis of care for hospital patients is the need each person presents in the course of his specific illness and his medical treatment.
T F   2. Close observation of a child's food attitudes and food and fluid intake provides an important basis for planning his hospital diet.
T F   3. Patients use various coping, or defense, mechanisms to relieve anxieties concerning the hospitalization experience.
T F   4. A problem in determining specific care needs of very young children is their inability to communicate their fears, pain, or desire adequately to help workers caring for them.
T F   5. A patient's housing situation has little relation to his illness or his continuing care.
T F   6. Most hospital patients retain their usual rights of decision and independent action and hence lose none of their self-identity.
T F   7. History-taking is an important skill to obtain needed information concerning the influence of past experience on present needs.
T F   8. A patient's social history is of little value in planning his diet.
T F   9. Once a diet treatment plan has been established, it should be followed continuously without any subsequent change.
T F 10. Normal nutrition needs are the basis for diet therapy.
T F 11. Personal goals of the patient do not relate to his diet therapy and instruction.

T F 12. A diet modified in energy value may be indicated for an obese patient.

T F 13. Ill patients with little appetite are stimulated more to eat by larger food portions.

T F 14. Observance of holidays and birthdays helps interest young and old patients in food and gives them needed support.

T F 15. Involvement of the patient's family in his diet therapy and teaching usually creates problems and is best avoided.

Multiple Choice

Circle the letter in front of the correct answer. Then check your answers by the test key (Appendix, p 270). Now compare all the possible answers for each item and write the following brief statements: (1) rationale for the correct answer and (2) why each one of the other responses is wrong.

1. Which of the following physical details help to determine a patient's nutritional needs?
   (1) age
   (2) sex
   (3) skin condition
   (4) symptoms of illness
   (5) disabilities
   a. 3, 4, and 5
   b. 1, 2, and 3
   c. 1, 4, and 5
   d. all of these

2. Factors that influence the patient's adjustment to hospitalization include:
   (1) age
   (2) degree of illness
   (3) kind of care received
   (4) ethnic cultural group background
   (5) financial resources
   a. 1, 2, and 3
   b. 3, 4, and 5
   c. all of these
   d. 2, 3, and 5

154

3.   A nutrition history should include which of the following nutritional data?
     (1)   general food habits
     (2)   food-buying practices
     (3)   cooking methods
     (4)   food likes and dislikes
     a.   1 and 3
     b.   all of these
     c.   1 and 4
     d.   2 and 4

4.   Knowledge of which of the following items is necessary for carrying out valid diet therapy for a hospitalized patient?
     (1)   the specific diet and its relation to the patient's disease
     (2)   foods affected by the diet modification
     (3)   mode of the hospital's food service and need of the patient for any eating aids
     (4)   the patient's response to the diet
     a.   1 and 2
     b.   2 and 4
     c.   all of these
     d.   2 and 3

5.   A therapeutic diet may be based on a specific nutrient modification. For example, a 30 g protein diet would include increased amounts of which of the following foods?
     a.   meat and fish
     b.   eggs and poultry
     c.   cheese and milk
     d.   fruits and vegetables

6.   A full liquid diet should include which of the following foods?
     (1)   ice cream
     (2)   custard
     (3)   cooked cereal
     (4)   applesauce
     a.   1 and 2
     b.   3 and 4
     c.   1 and 4
     d.   2 and 3

155

7.   Which of the following patient care actions would be helpful to a disabled patient who needs assistance in eating?
      (1)   learning the extent of his disability and encouraging him to do as much of the feeding as he can for himself
      (2)   feeding the patient completely, regardless of his problem, since it saves him time and energy
      (3)   hurrying the feeding to get in as much food as possible before his appetite wanes
      (4)   sitting comfortably by the patient's bed and offering him mouthfuls of food, with ample time between for him to chew, swallow, and rest as needed
      a.   2 and 3
      b.   1 and 4
      c.   1 and 3
      d.   2 and 4

Learning Activities

Group Project: Role of the Registered Dietitian (RD) in Patient Care

    Assign members of the class, perhaps by twos to visit a number of different-sized hospitals available in the surrounding community. If possible, include a large medical center, a smaller community hospital, and a community health center.

    At each of these medical care facilities arrange to interview various dietitians concerning their roles in patient care. Include the following types of dietitians in your interviews if possible:
      1.   clinic dietitian in outpatient setting
      2.   administrative dietitian or dietary department director
      3.   clinical or patient care dietitian in hospital
      4.   consulting dietitian to nursing homes
      5.   nutritionist in a community health center
      6.   clinical nutrition specialist in private practice
Include the following points in your interview:
      1.   What system of food service is being used?
      2.   What is the relation of the dietitian to other patient care personnel such as physicians, nurses, social workers, and others?
      3.   What types of activities does she conduct with patients and staff personnel?
      4.   What relationship does she have with the hospital administrator?
Observe tray service in the hospital. Note the form of tray service used, the types of diets being served, and the nature of the foods being used in each.

Individual Observations: Nutrition Histories in Care of Patients on Therapeutic Diets

    Make an appointment with a hospital dietitian and arrange to accompany her on ward rounds to visit newly admitted hospitalized patients. Observe her technique in taking a nutrition history as a basis for planning care for the patient while he is in the

156

hospital and for making suggestions for his diet when he goes home. Discuss with her afterward any selected patients, in terms of disease and relation of diet therapy and any individual personal situations influencing the diet plan.

With the clinical dietitian, review a selected number of hospital patients' charts to determine what, if any, routine nutrition assessment is done on administration and followed during the hospitalization. On the basis of your findings, what recommendations would you make?

Arrange a visit with an outpatient clinic dietitian at the medical center or with a consulting nutritionist in private practice in the community. Observe her taking a nutrition history with a medical patient. Afterward discuss with her your observations. Under her guidance and observation, conduct a diet history yourself, if it is suitable in this situation. Then discuss your experience with the dietitian.

Compare experiences of class members in class reports of these experiences. What factors were brought out in the various nutrition histories that provided useful information for planning the patient's diet? What needs were not brought out that you think should have been included?

Individual Project: Feeding Disabled Patients or Children

Arrange with any available health care facility in the community to assist in the feeding of a disabled patient or small child. Select a variety of hospital or community care settings such as nursing homes or hospitals.

Observe the patient's reaction and attitudes expressed toward the food. What degree of feeding assistance did the patient require? What plan of feeding assistance did you find worked best? If a rehabilitation hospital is available in your community, visit the center and observe the variety of devices that may be used to assist the patients in feeding themselves. If you are visiting a pediatric ward, compare the reactions of various children to the food being served them.

Current Nutrition Issues

Read carefully the *Issues and Answers* article, "Selecting Computer Nutrient-Calculation Software" (*Essentials of Nutrition and Diet Therapy*, ed 6, p 320; *Nutrition and Diet Therapy*, ed 7, p 475). Consider these inquiry questions:

1.   Identify some of the advantages you have found in using modern computer analysis for evaluation of nutritional data.

157

2.   Why is the quality of the nutrient database fundamental to the quality of the resulting nutrient/energy analysis?   What is the major source of the nutrient/energy database for most available assessment programs in the U.S.? Why is this source a valuable one?

3.   What important questions should you ask about the database in any software package you were considering for purchase? Give your reasons in each case.

Chapter 17
DRUG-NUTRIENT INTERACTION

Chapter Focus

The relation of food and nutrients to drug actions in the body is complex. Basic knowledge of these interactions is essential for both practitioner and patient to make wise and effective use of drug and nutritional therapy.

Summary-Review Quiz

Fill in the blanks below with the appropriate number and word(s) from the list following each section. Each numbered word or phrase is used; some may be used more than once. When you have completed all the sections, check your answers for each blank by the test key (Appendix, p 271). Correct any mistakes and then review the entire chapter summary.

1.   Concerned _____ and the public have come to view our _____ society with alarm. American medicine is _____, with a large _____ array of drugs being _____ by physicians. Also, in response to expensive corporate marketing, American _____ purchase large volumes of _____ drugs over the counter.

2.   Clinicians and _____ indicate that a _____ of the marketed drugs would take care of most _____ problems. In many cases most drugs are only _____ of a basic _____ drug sold under a variety of trade names, the so-called "me too" drugs. Usually use of the _____ drug can be a means of cost control.

3.   Much of this _____ problem in American medicine results from an increasingly complex and _____ practice, caused by a rapidly advancing _____ . Each _____ or discipline can easily become _____ from other interacting factors such as a patient's _____ and not realize a particular drug's impact. A _____ approach helps to prevent such _____ problems.

1. drug-oriented	8. isolated	15. nutritional state
2. consumers	9. overmedicated	16. practitioners
3. general medical	10. slight variations	17. technology
4. nutrient-drug interaction	11. health organizations	18. small fraction
5. specialized	12. specialist	19. multiple drug use
6. nonprescription	13. confusing	20. prescribed
7. team	14. generic	

4.   Any age person may risk harmful _____ but _____ are particularly at risk because of (1) use of _____ for longer periods of time to control _____ and (2) errors in _____ from _____, lack of _____ or _____.

5.   General _____ may also result from _____. The greater number of _____ using during hospitalization may interfere with _____ and _____ for use by the body.

1. chronic diseases	5. hospital malnutrition	9. drug-nutrient interactions
2. drug information	6. self-care	10. drugs and procedures
3. elderly persons	7. food intake	11. illness
4. nutrient availability	8. mental confusion	12. more drugs

6.   Drugs may affect food _____ by: (1) increasing or decreasing _____, (2) causing _____, (3) creating _____, or (4) increasing _____ with nondigestible fiber.

7.   Drugs may also influence nutrient _____ by: (1) increasing or decreasing _____, (2) causing loss of _____ by inducing _____ losses or increasing _____ excretion, (3) causing loss of _____ by action as a _____, or (4) causing special adverse reactions such as inhibiting specific _____ or inducing _____.

1. dietary bulk	6. hypoglycemia	11. vitamins
2. metabolic antagonist	7. availability	12. intake
3. appetite	8. nausea	13. gastrointestinal
4. minerals	9. cell enzyme actions	14. taste changes
5. renal	10. absorption	

8.   Food and nutrients influence drug _____ in the body by: (1) increasing or decreasing _____ and (2) hindering or facilitating _____ and _____.

9.   Food may affect the _____ of a drug by influencing (1) the rate at which the drug goes into _____, (2) the _____ rate, and (3) the _____ rate.

10.   Aspirin use is hindered by the presence of _____ in the stomach causing (1) decreased _____ rate and (2) faster _____ time. This common drug is best taken on an _____ with a full glass of _____.

1. absorption	5. drug absorption	9. visceral blood flow
2. metabolism	6. cold water	10. action
3. dissolution	7. solution	11. food
4. stomach emptying	8. empty stomach	12. drug distribution

Discussion Questions

1.   Why do you think such a large volume of drugs are used--and abused--in this country? What solutions can you suggest for the problem of multiple drug use?

2.   How many drugs affect our nutritional status? Give some examples.

3.   What is meant by the *first-pass* mechanism of drug absorption?

4.   Why would gastric emptying time have an effect on utilization of a drug? How does the composition of a meal influence the time it stays in the stomach?

5.   How does food affect drug distribution and metabolism? Give some examples.

Self-Test Questions

True-False
      Circle the "T" if a statement is true and write a brief rationale for its accuracy. If it is false, circle the "F" and write the correct statement.

T F 1.   Amphetamines are widely used as appetite depressants in the treatment of obesity.
T F 2.   The chelating agent D-penicillamine used in treatment of rheumatoid arthritis causes a loss of taste and hence anorexia.
T F 3.   The bulking agent methyl cellulose may interfere with absorption of nutrients.
T F 4.   The gastric antisecretory agent, cimetidine, decreases nutrient absorption.
T F 5.   Alcohol abuse causes malabsorption of thiamin and folic acid.
T F 6.   The antibiotic, neomycin, causes a primary malabsorption and deficiency of calcium.
T F 7.   Salicylates such as aspirin can induce an iron deficiency.
T F 8.   Aspirin should never be taken on an empty stomach.
T F 9.   Women using oral contraceptive agents should take increased amounts of vitamin B_6.

T F   10.   The method of cooking foods may alter the rate of metabolism of drugs being used.

Multiple Choice

Circle the letter in front of the correct answer. Then check your answers by the test key (Appendix, p 272). Now compare all the possible answers for each item and write the following brief statements: (1) rationale for the correct answer and (2) why each one of the other responses is wrong.

1.   Persons in which of the following age groups have a higher risk of harmful drug or drug-nutrient interactions?
   a.   infants and young children
   b.   adolescents
   c.   young adults
   d.   elderly adults

2.   Methyl cellulose decreases appetite through which of the following actions?
   a.   binds nutrients and prevents their absorption
   b.   adds bulk to the diet
   c.   slows passage of food from stomach
   d.   causes a loss of taste and hence anorexia

3.   Which one of the following drugs benefits nutritional status by increasing nutrient absorption?
   a.   cimetidine
   b.   neomycin
   c.   colchicine
   d.   methotrexate

4.   Diuretic agents intentionally used to reduce levels of tissue water and sodium may also interfere with normal heart action through dangerous loss of what other mineral?
   a.   calcium
   b.   phosphate
   c.   potassium
   d.   zinc

5.   The anticoagulant agent, coumarin, achieves its effect by acting as a metabolic antagonist to which of the following nutrients?
   a.   vitamin E
   b.   iron
   c.   calcium
   d.   vitamin K

Learning Activities

Individual Project: Analysis of a Patient's Drug Use

Select an elderly medical or surgical patient in the hospital or in a clinic who is being treated for any chronic illness or condition. Interview this patient, taking both a nutrition and a drug history in relation to medical care. Include both prescription and nonprescription drugs.

Identify all drugs being used in terms of:
1. chemical or generic name
2. trade name and drug company producing it
3. cost—compare generic and trade product
4. dosage and instructions for use
5. main physiologic action
6. any food or nutrient interactions
7. side effects
8. patient's knowledge of each drug according to its full nature and use

Plan a follow-up teaching visit with the patient to review all drugs used as outlined above.

Individual of Group Project: Drug Products Survey

Plan a visit to a community pharmacy. Study a number of nonprescription drug products, reading label information and checking cost. Note particularly those drugs having food or nutrient interactions, such as:
1. laxatives
2. appetite suppressants
3. antacids
4. food supplements or special formulas
5. vitamins, minerals
6. analgesics
7. allergy relief products

Evaluate these products and discuss your findings in class.

Individual Project: Interview with Pharmacist

Plan ahead an appropriate time to interview a pharmacist about the role of the pharmacist or pharmacologist on a medical or health care team. Discuss their work with customers, clients, or patients in relation to drug education, both nonprescription and prescription drugs, and use of generic and trade drugs with comparative costs. Also discuss selected drugs having food or nutrient interactions and andy practice in counseling patients about proper use. Particularly review any attention to elderly patients on multiple drugs.

Report your findings in class discussion, comparing your interview results with those of other class members.

Individual Project; "What's in Your Medicine Chest?"

Open your own medicine chest at home. Review carefully all drug items and list everything you find. Identify each item as outlined above. How many are in current use? How many are outdated?

Dispose of all outdated items appropriately. Indicate reasons for continued use of other items. What instructions for their use did you receive? From what source? Evaluate your own experience with medications accordingly.

Current Nutrition Issues

Read carefully the *Issues and Answers* article, "The Calming of America" (*Essentials of Nutrition and Diet Therapy*, ed 6, p 332); *Nutrition and Diet Therapy*, ed 7, p 487). Consider these inquiry questions:

1. Why do you think Americans use such a large amount of tranquilizers? Why are they so easily abused?

2. What are some of the effects of the aggressive marketing program used by the drug company producing the psychoactive drug Valium?

3. How do these psychoactive drugs act in the body?

4. What possible interactions with food and alcohol may occur? Why is such a drug especially dangerous during pregnancy and lactation?

Chapter 18
FEEDING METHODS: ENTERAL AND PARENTERAL NUTRITION

Chapter Focus

In severe hypermetabolic illness or injury, alternate means of securing essential nutrition support through enteral or parenteral feeding methods is often required. When the gastrointestinal tract can be used, enteral feeding by oral supplementation or special formulas by tube feeding is often the method of choice. If the gastrointestinal tract cannot be used, concentrated parenteral solutions of needed nutrients can be fed directly into central or peripheral veins to meet critical requirements.

Summary-Review Quiz

Fill in the blanks below with the appropriate number and word(s) from the list following each section. Each numbered word or phrase is used; some may be used more than once. When you have completed all the sections, check your answers for each blank by the test key (Appendix, p 272). Correct any mistakes and then review the entire chapter summary.

1. Significant protein-energy _____ is a serious concern among _____ patients. Particularly at risk are persons with underlying _____ or _____. Especially vulnerable are _____.

2. In cases of a functional _____, nutrition support by _____ methods provides the front line of restoring optimal nutritional status. Major concerns center on the _____ for each patient's specific _____, the preferred method of _____, and management of possible _____.

3. The two possible routes of _____ nutrition support are oral supplementation or _____. Careful _____ of each hospital patient at admission identifies persons at risk of potential _____. Individual nutritional needs are based on the underlying _____ with added _____ according to the patient's clinical stress due to disease, _____, _____, or sepsis.

4. A basic factor indicating need of nutritional support for medical-surgical patients is inability to eat for more than _____. After patient identification of nutritional need and a functional _____, choices of _____ and _____ system follow.

1. surgery
2. tube-related complications
3. appropriate formula
4. disease or injury
5. 7 to 10 days
6. enteral
7. metabolic activity factors (MAT)

8. chronic disease
9. surgical and medical
10. tube feeding
11. traumatic injury
12. formula delivery
13. gastrointestinal tract
14. disease state

15. elderly persons
16. malnutrition
17. nutrition assessment

5.   Problems of _____, _____, and digestion and absorption occur with the use of home-prepared _____, so they are rarely used now. In comparison, today's development of _____ provides _____ solutions suitable for the more comfortable current _____.

6.   The components in modern _____ ensure a fixed _____ in an _____ form. Carbohydrates are provided as small _____, mainly _____, or hydrolyzed intermediate products such as _____ or short-chain _____ of 3-10 glucose units. The disaccharide _____ is often deleted in _____ formulas due to poor tolerance.

7.   Three major forms of protein used in _____ formulas are: (1) intact forms of protein isolates such as _____ from milk; (2) hydrolyzed products such as small _____ and free _____; and (3) easily absorbed _____.

8.   Fat is supplied as (1) _____ in milk formulas; (2) _____ from corn, soy, or safflower oils, which are rich sources of the essential fatty acid _____; and (3) specially produced _____ , mono- and diglycerides, and lecithin. Current research is developing new alternate _____ from various combinations of _____ fatty acids and the larger _____ fatty acids. Then for complete nutrition, standard _____ add sufficient _____ to meet needs for increased _____ work.

1. simple sugars	10. enteral nutrition support	19. lactose
2. structured lipids	11. sterile homogenized	20. oligosaccharides
3. metabolic	12. omega-3	21. small-bore flexible feeding tubes
4. amino acids	13. intact or predigested	22. crystalline amino acids
5. linoleic acid	14. vitamins and minerals	23. physical form
6. short- and medium chain	15. vegetable oils	24. nutrient composition
7. glucose polysaccharides	16. safety	25. blender-mixed formulas
8. commercial formulas	17. lactalbumin and casein	26. medium-chain triglyceride (MCT)
9. peptides	18. butterfat	27. glucose

9.   The feeding equipment for enteral nutrition delivery systems involves _____, _____, and often an _____. For short-term therapy, small soft modern _____ may be placed into the _____, or lower down through the _____ into the _____ of the small intestine.

10.   For long-term therapy, surgical tube placement by _____ at progressive points along the _____ are used to deliver the formula. Progressively, any one of three surgical placement procedures may be used: (1) _____, (2) _____, or (3) _____.

11.   Monitoring the tube-fed patient includes nursing observations such as (1) gastric _____; (2) signs of abdominal _____; and (3) vital signs of _____. Attending nurses also monitor the formula _____ and record _____ of formula and fluid, and report _____ to the formula.

12.   The nutrition support team clinical dietitian monitors _____, state of _____, and _____, using assessment protocols, and _____ the formula according to individual need. Careful _____ of all observations, corrective actions, and follow-up by _____ involved in enteral nutrition tube-feeding is essential.

166

1. stomach
2. flow rate
3. jejunostomy
4. adjusts or recalculates
5. formula tolerance
6. distention or bloating
7. enterostomies
8. nutrition support team members
9. infusion pump
10. nutritional status
11. gastrostomy
12. formula containers
13. temperature, pulse, respiration (TPR)
14. gastrointestinal tract
15. individual patient responses
16. nasoenteric tubes
17. documentation
18. feeding tubes
19. hydration
20. pyloric valve
21. esophagostomy
22. residuals or emptying rate
23. intake and output
24. duodenum or jejunum

13.   When the gastrointestinal tract cannot be used, _____ is used to meet nutritional needs by feeding _____ of basic nutrients directly into a _____ for long periods of time, or feeding _____ into _____ for shorter periods of time.

14.   The lengthy and complete sustaining of individual _____ to meet the hypermetabolic demands of _____ through intravenous feeding has been termed _____. Three factors govern decisions about use of this complete feeding method: (1) availability of the _____, (2) degree of _____, and (3) degree of _____ or catabolism.

15.   Initial baseline _____ provides the necessary data for: (1) _____ requiring special therapy, (2) _____ for energy and nutrients, and (3) determining the _____ to meet needs. The ongoing monitoring of _____ helps maintain _____ and avoids _____.

16.   Nutrient components of a _____ include: (1) protein-nitrogen source—essential and nonessential _____, usually standard 8.5% solution; (2) nonprotein energy source (kcalories)—_____, usually standard hypertonic 50% solution, and a _____ for concentrated energy and the _____, linoleic acid; (3) _____ for fluid and acid-base balance and other metabolic activities; (4) _____ for protein-energy metabolism; and (5) _____ for special individual metabolic functions.

1. nutritional requirements
2. total parenteral nutrition (TPN)
3. identifying patients
4. nutritional status
5. metabolic complications
6. malnutrition
7. small peripheral veins
8. optimal therapy
9. calculating requirements
10. crystalline amino acids
11. parenteral nutrition
12. lipid emulsion
13. gastrointestinal tract
14. large central vein
15. trace elements
16. essential fatty acid
17. concentrated hypertonic solutions
18. electrolytes
19. nutrition assessment
20. vitamins
21. less concentrated solution
22. specific formula
23. debilitating illness or injury
24. TPN solution
25. glucose
26. hypermetabolism

Discussion Questions

1. How do physical properties of enteral formulas create tolerance problems? What is the most common of these problems? Why?

2. What are "medical foods"? Why has there been difficulty in defining these nutritional formulas? Give some examples of these special formulas to meet particular medical problems.

3. How do modular enteral formulas differ from standard formulas? In what patient situations would they be used? How are they developed and prepared?

4. Compare the three enterostomies for surgical placement of feeding tubes in terms of situations in which each would be the procedure of choice.

Self-Test Questions

<u>True-False</u>

Circle the "T" if a statement is true and write a brief rationale for its accuracy. If it is false, circle the "F" and write the correct statement.

T F 1. The full effectiveness of enteral nutrition support (ENS), even by tube-feeding, has yet to be completely established.

T F 2. Since its attention over the past decade, protein-energy malnutrition is no longer a serious concern in hospitalized medical and surgical patients.

T F 3. Tube-feeding is the wisest initial choice for ENS because it can deliver a more concentrated supply of nutrients.

T F 4. Blender-mixed oral or tube-fed formulas are commonly used because regular foods bring emotional comfort.

T F 5. The major role of fat in enteral formulas is to supply a concentrated energy source to meet hypermetabolic demands.

T F 6. When the gastrointestinal tract cannot be used, parenteral nutrition support methods can deliver concentrated nutrient solutions directly into a large central vein or a less concentrated solution into smaller peripheral veins.

T F 7. Among biochemical tests for nutrition assessment and monitoring of patients on total parenteral nutrition (TPN), a measure of the plasma protein *prealbumin (PAB)* is the most sensitive marker of current status because of its short half-life of only two days.

T F 8. Generally clinicians caring for TPN patients give little value to the constant kcalorie intake but look more to regular measures of protein-nitrogen adequacy.

T F 9. Lipid emulsions used in TPN therapy must be fed separately from the basic glucose-amino acid solution.

T F 10. Needed trace elements are also easily administered in the entire TPN solution.

<u>Multiple Choice</u>

Circle the letter in front of the correct answer. Then check your answers by the test key (Appendix, p 274). Now compare all the possible answers for each item and write the following brief statements: (1) rationale for the correct answer, and (2) why each one of the other responses is wrong.

1. In TPN therapy, following nutrition support team protocols and monitoring results, the specialist team member carrying major responsibility for assessing the patient's nutritional status, calculating energy-nutrient needs, and formulating appropriate solutions to meet these needs is the:
    a. physician
    b. clinical dietitian
    c. nurse
    d. pharmacist

2. Strict aseptic technique and infection control throughout the entire TPN administration is the major responsibility of:
    a. the pharmacist who prepares the TPN solution
    b. the surgeon who inserts and places the venous catheter
    c. the nurse who cares for the catheter site and all external equipment and administers the solution
    d. all of these support team members
3. Home enteral tube-feeding provides a useful continuing means of nutrition support because it:
    a. meets physiologic needs
    b. provides a safe and relatively simple system to manage
    c. costs far less than TPN
    d. all of the above
4. Education of the patient and family for home tube-feeding is best done by the nutrition support team:
    a. physician
    b. nurse
    c. clinical dietitian and nurse together
    d. pharmacist
5. Home parenteral nutrition support (TPN) provides complete continuing nourishment that is:
    a. easily administered by all TPN patients and families
    b. used successfully by carefully selected and well-trained patients
    c. relatively inexpensive for long-term use
    d. a difficult and limited means of mobility

Learning Activities

Individual Project: Roles of Nutrition Support Team Members

Obtain a copy of the operational protocol of the special nutrition support program in your hospital. Note particularly the standard procedures and roles of the team clinical dietitian, nurse, pharmacist, and physician. How was your hospital's particular guiding document developed and approved?

Interview the clinical dietitian team member and identify this specialist's specific roles in nutrition assessment, nutrient-energy determinations, the tube-feeding formula or TPN solution development.

Interview the team nurse to identify specific responsibilities in administering the tube-fed formula or intravenous TPN solution, the types of equipment used for each method, maintaining strict infection control, and providing individual patient support. If possible arrange a patient visit with the nurse to observe a feeding.

Interview the team pharmacist to identify specific responsibilities in the special nutrition support program. If possible, arrange a visit to the hospital pharmacy to observe the special aseptic methods and equipment used in mixing the TPN solution. Note the products used to supply each nutrient component in the prescribed strengths and amounts.

In all cases, discuss with each team specialist their specific charting of observations, actions, and recommendations concerning the nutrition support therapy in the patient's medical record. Also discuss team operations in terms of regular meetings, agenda, and clinical case conferences of patients.

Individual or Small Group Project: Home Nutrition Support

Discuss with the nutrition support dietitian and nurse the procedures followed in educating the patient and family for continuing the nutrition support program at home after hospital discharge. What is the content of this learning and how is the instruction carried out before discharge? What follow-up reinforcement and continuing education occurs? If possible, arrange to accompany the dietitian and/or nurse on a follow-up home visit, or to observe a patient's return visit to the out-patient clinic. Report these clinical experiences to the class.

Group Project: Comparison of Commercial Nutrition Formulas

Arrange with the clinical dietitian to hold a taste-testing session for comparing oral and tube-fed enteral nutrition support formulas. Note the nutrient-energy formulation of each standard or special formula, their designated use, and comparative costs. How are these products marketed by the companies producing them?

Current Nutrition Issues

Read carefully the *Issues and Answers* article, "Troubleshooting Diarrhea in Tube-Fed Patients: A Costly Chase" (*Essentials of Nutrition and Diet Therapy*, ed 6, p 351; *Nutrition and Diet Therapy*, ed 7, p 503). Consider these inquiry questions:

1.   Why is the problem of diarrhea frequent in tube-fed patients? Why is it sometimes a difficult problem to solve?

2.   What possible problems may related to formula factors? How may they be solved?

3.   How may bacterial contamination occur in the formula or feeding system? What solutions to this problem can you suggest?

4.   What role may the patient's condition play in the development of diarrhea?

5.   How may medications be involved? In the case of Max, how do you think the costly chase for the culprit may have been avoided?

Chapter 19
GASTROINTESTINAL PROBLEMS

Chapter Focus

Nutritional support for persons with gastrointestinal problems must focus on individual needs, given the functional capacity of the person to handle food. Depending on this capacity in any part of the gastrointestinal tract or its accessory organs, the food forms and diet management will need to be varied to meet nutritional therapy needs.

Summary-Review Quiz

Fill in the blanks below with the appropriate number and word(s) from the list following each section. Each numbered word or phrase is used; some may be used more than once. When you have completed all the sections, check your answers for each blank by the test key (Appendix, p 275). Correct any mistakes and then review the entire chapter summary.

1.   Diet therapy used in diseases of the gastrointestinal system relates specifically to the _____ of the affected organs and the degree of _____ with that normal _____.

2.   The functioning of the gastrointestinal tract mirrors the total _____ of the individual and personal _____ influences. Thus diet therapy for gastrointestinal problems will concern not only (1) _____ associated with digestion, (2) _____ that moves and mixes the food mass, and (3) the _____ lining the intestine, but also (4) the _____ and his own stress-coping responses. All of the factors must be considered in planning effective _____.

1. function
2. chemical secretions
3. physical and psychosocial
4. person
5. disease interference

6. absorbing mucosal surfaces
7. nutritional therapy
8. normal physiology
9. muscle activity
10. life situation

3.   Problems in the _____ involve _____ and functions of this entrance to the gastrointestinal tract. The most prevalent mouth problem in young children is _____. Factors that work together to cause this widespread problem are the _____ of the child's _____, the oral _____ in the dental plaque, and frequent use of _____ foods. An effective control agent has proved to be _____. Problems with ill-fitting _____ or injury such as a _____ interfere with proper chewing and use of _____. Defects in operation of the lower esophageal sphincter muscles cause problems of (1) _____, muscle spasm, or (2) _____, reflux of gastric acid. Also, at the juncture of the

esophagus and the stomach a _____ hinders normal food passage and causes much discomfort.

1. gastroesophageal reflux disease	6. structures	11. mouth and esophagus
2. bacteria	7. solid foods	12. fluoride
3. fractured jaw	8. shape and structure	13. achalasia
4. teeth	9. frequent snack	14. dental caries
5. hiatal hernia	10. dentures	

4.   Problems in the stomach and duodenum center mainly around various degrees of _____. Although the basic cause is unclear, two factors involved are gastric secretion of _____ and the degree of _____. The _____ factor may also contribute to ulcer development but the basic lesions result from _____ of mucosal tissue. Thus successful therapy must focus on the _____ with the ulcer. In general, a _____, based on three well-balanced regular meals a day with infrequent snacks, is preferred, with individual _____ and the degree of _____ being the guides.

5.   Problems in the intestines include several general functional disorders. One of these, _____, results from excessive or inadequate action of the colon muscles with consequent discomfort and _____. Other similar bowel problems include _____, often a reflection of other difficulties, and _____, which when prolonged in infants can cause serious _____ losses. Diet treatment for these functional problems usually involves attention to intake of _____ and _____.

1. psychologic	7. constipation	13. changes in bowel habits
2. irritable bowel syndrome	8. disease activity	14. fluid and electrolyte
3. food tolerances	9. acid erosion	15. tissue resistance
4. person	10. water	16. liberal diet approach
5. dietary fiber	11. diarrhea	
6. acid and pepsin	12. peptic ulcer disease	

6.   Organic diseases of the intestine may be due to (1) anatomic changes as in _____, (2) problems of _____ as in celiac-sprue, or (3)_____ changes as in Crohn's disease or ulcerative colitis, similar conditions included in general _____.

7.   The colon disease _____ is a condition in which small _____ develop at weakened muscle points. Inflammation at these points causes _____ with constricting muscle action and resulting pain, gastrointestinal disturbances, and fever. Treatment centers on an increase in _____ to prevent painful _____, reduce symptoms, and allow _____.

1. celiac-sprue
2. diverticulitis
3. inflammatory bowel disease
4. dietary fiber
5. malabsorption
6. pouches
7. healing
8. diverticulosis
9. bowel contractions
10. infectious mucosal tissue

8.   Problems of _____ such as _____ lead to general _____ from loss of numerous _____ and the characteristic frequent _____ stools. The underlying causative agent is _____, a protein found in certain grains, mainly _____. Thus therapy is based on a _____ diet to remove most of this offending agent, with food _____ modified according to the individual need.

9.   The conditions of _____ result from lesions of the mucous membrane of the intestine, with a characteristic continuous, chronic, _____ diarrhea and gross losses of many _____. Nutritional therapy centers on vigorous replacement of _____, especially _____ needed for tissue healing, sufficient _____ for energy demands and to spare _____, increased _____, and _____ adjustment according to individual healing progress and degree of mucosal tissue _____. Repeated surgical resections for continued disease result in _____, severe dysfunction of the remaining portion of the organ.

1. nutrients
2. progressive texture
3. celiac-sprue
4. bloody
5. protein
6. gluten-free
7. minerals and vitamins
8. malnutrition
9. inflammatory bowel disease
10. gluten
11. nutrient losses
12. texture
13. wheat
14. malabsorption
15. inflammation
16. bulky and fatty
17. kcalories
18. short bowel syndrome

10.   Various food intolerances may also cause problems. These may be metabolic problems of _____ origin, such as _____ or _____, both of which, if not _____ and treated, can cause severe _____. In each case the _____ not tolerated must be _____ in the child's food and careful management of the total diet continued. In cases of _____ the nutrient involved is the amino acid _____. In cases of _____ the nutrient involved is the milk sugar, _____, from which the offending simple sugar _____ is derived during digestion.

1. screened at birth
2. specific nutrient
3. lactose
4. phenylketonuria
5. galactosemia
6. phenylalanine
7. mental retardation
8. galactose
9. genetic
10. controlled

11.   A similar _____ problem, but caused by a different missing enzyme, _____, is _____ that occurs mainly in _____, Oriental, and American Indian populations. In affected persons, milk causes _____ with resulting fluid loss and _____.

12.   Problems of _____, a disorder of the immune system, are caused by a number of agents to which an affected person is highly sensitive. The foods most commonly involved are _____, egg, and wheat. Diet therapy consists of strict removal of the _____ from the diet.

1. Black
2. milk
3. dehydration

4. specific allergen
5. lactase
6. food allergy

7. diarrhea
8. genetic
9. lactose intolerance

13.   Disease in the three accessory organs to the gastrointestinal tract, the liver, _____, and pancreas, may also cause metabolic and gastrointestinal problems. Treatment for the liver disease _____, especially the advanced form of _____, centers mainly on the use of increased _____ according to individual tolerance. In the complication stage of _____, however, this key nutrient must be _____.

14.   In gallbladder disease the specific nutrient modification involved in diet therapy is _____ because this organ provides _____ to assist in _____ of this nutrient. The general treatment therefore includes attention to the amount of _____.

1. fat
2. digestion and absorption
3. hepatitis
4. dietary fat

5. decreased
6. cirrhosis
7. bile
8. hepatic encephalopathy

9. gallbladder
10. protein

15.   Cystic fibrosis is a generalized _____ disease of children, which can be screened prenatally or at birth since recent discovery of the _____, but until a cure is found generally causes death by _____. The disease affects secretions in many tissues and organs, especially the _____ and lungs. Pancreatic _____ are decreased or absent, causing pancreatic insufficiency due to mucus-clogged ducts. As a result, foods digested by these _____ cannot be used properly by the body. There is subsequent _____ of these food components and the characteristic diarrhea with _____ stools containing much _____ food, resulting in extensive _____.   Current management consists of _____, combined with comprehensive initial and ongoing _____ and aggressive nutritional therapy on any one of five diagnosed levels according to individual _____.   The diet therapy centers on correcting the large _____, especially of _____ needed for tissue growth.

175

1. malabsorption
2. undigested
3. protein
4. enzymes
5. assessment
6. nutrient losses
7. hereditary
8. enzyme replacement
9. bulky and fatty
10. pancreas
11. malnutrition
12. nutritional status
13. young adult years
14. causative gene

Discussion Questions

1.   How do you account for the large incidence of dental caries in young children? What would you include in a treatment program? Why?

2.   When explaining the current use of a regular diet for a patient with peptic ulcer disease, how would you explain the change from traditional restricted diet approaches used in the past?

3.   Describe the basic disease problem in inflammatory bowel disease. Relate this disease and its nutritional therapy to interference with normal functioning of the intestine. How would you plan a diet for such a patient? What foods would you use? What teaching would this patient need?

4.   What role does fiber play in diverticular disease? What possible relation may fiber have in the treatment of other gastrointestinal problems?

5.   What are the principles of diet therapy in the spectrum of liver disease states—hepatitis, cirrhosis, and hepatic encephalopathy? What is the key nutrient involved? Why? How is it modified? How would you plan a diet for a patient with the advanced hepatitis state of cirrhosis?

Self-Test Questions

<u>True-False</u>

Circle the "T" if a statement is true and write a brief rationale for its accuracy. If it is false, circle the "F" and write the correct statement.

T F 1. Fluoridation of a community water supply greatly reduces the incidence of dental caries.

T F 2. A mechanical soft diet may be indicated for patients with dental problems.

T F 3. Lying down after eating helps a person with a hiatal hernia to relieve discomfort.

T F 4. The fundamental cause of peptic ulcer is not completely understood.

T F 5. The ulcer-prone individual tends to be relaxed and noncompetitive.

T F 6. Peptic ulcer pain is reduced when the stomach is empty of food because the organ can then rest and heal.

T F 7. Studies of patients with peptic ulcer disease indicate that bland foods do not increase the rate of healing.

T F 8. A low-residue diet is advocated for treatment of diverticulosis.

T F 9. Infectious diarrhea in infants is seldom a serious problem.

T F 10. All food sources of the grains wheat, rye, oats, buckwheat, and barley must be omitted on the gluten-free diet for sprue or celiac disease.

T F 11. PKU is a genetic disease caused by the absence of a specific cell enzyme needed to metabolize the amino acid phenylalanine.

T F 12. Since phenylalanine is a nonessential amino acid, it can be totally removed from the infant's diet.

T F 13. A diet for a child with galactosemia would omit all foods containing lactose.

T F 14. Soybean preparations are often used for children allergic to milk.

<u>Multiple Choice</u>

Circle the letter in front of the correct answer. Then check your answers by the test key (Appendix, p 276). Now compare all the possible answers for each item and write the following brief statements: (1) rationale for the correct answer and (2) why each one of the other responses is incorrect.

1. Basic treatment for peptic ulcer disease includes:
    (1) drugs to control gastric secretion and help buffer stomach acid
    (2) use of only bland foods to buffer acid secretions
    (3) withholding cold food to avoid tissue irritation and bleeding
    (4) three regular well-balanced meals a day with infrequent snacks to control gastric acid secretion and promote healing
    a.   3 and 4
    b.   2 and 3
    c.   1 and 4
    d.   1 and 3

2. The sequence of treatment for prolonged infectious diarrhea in children includes:
    (1) initial intravenous fluid and electrolyte replacement
    (2) oral fluids when tolerated, including glucose and balanced salt solutions
    (3) milk mixtures or milk substitutes to increase protein intake
    (4) kilocalories increased to normal requirement as soon as possible
    a.   2 and 3
    b.   3 and 4
    c.   1 and 4
    d.   all of these

3. In a gluten-free diet for celiac-sprue, which of the following foods would be omitted?
    a.   eggs
    b.   milk
    c.   rice
    d.   saltine crackers

4. The symptoms of anemia in malabsorption diseases are caused by poor absorption of:
    a.   vitamin K
    b.   iron and folic acid
    c.   calcium and phosphorus
    d.   fats

5. Clinical symptoms associated with the nutritional problems of ulcerative colitis include:
    (1) loss of appetite
    (2) edema
    (3) anemia
    (4) negative nitrogen balance
    (5) weight loss
    a.   1 and 5
    b.   2 and 4
    c.   4 and 5
    d.   all of these

6. Diet therapy for ulcerative colitis includes:
    (1) decreased kcalories to avoid food irritation
    (2) increased protein to replace losses and promote healing
    (3) increased amounts of milk to soothe the inflamed tissue
    (4) increased minerals and vitamins, usually including supplements, to replace losses and assist healing
    a. 1 and 2
    b. 3 and 4
    c. 2 and 4
    d. 1 and 3
7. Lactose intolerance in certain population groups is caused by a genetic deficiency of the enzyme:
    a. sucrase
    b. pepsin
    c. lactase
    d. maltase
8. Treatment for hepatic encephalopathy includes:
    a. increased protein to aid healing of liver cells
    b. decreased protein to reduce blood ammonia levels
    c. decreased kilocalories to reduce the metabolic load
    d. increased fluid intake to stimulate output
9. The multiple metabolic problems of the advanced state of liver disease, cirrhosis, are best treated by:
    (1) protein according to tolerance, to help heal liver tissue
    (2) sodium restriction to help control ascites
    (3) smooth texture to avoid irritation and possible rupture of swollen esophageal blood vessels
    (4) increased carbohydrate to provide energy
    a. 2 and 3
    b. 1 and 4
    c. all of these
    d. 2 and 4
10. Which of the following foods may be restricted in the diet of a surgery patient who has had a cholecystectomy?
    a. bacon
    b. skimmed milk
    c. bread
    d. fruit

Learning Activities

Situational Problem: Paul's Adaptation to Cystic Fibrosis
    Paul is a 12-year-old boy with cystic fibrosis. He is presently hospitalized with pneumonia and has difficulty breathing. He is a thin child with little muscle development

and tires easily, although he has a large appetite. His stools are large and frequent and contain undigested food material. His extensive assessment currently indicated a need for Level II nutritional therapy.

1. What is cystic fibrosis? Account for the clinical effects produced by the disease process as evidenced by Paul's appearance and symptoms.

2. What are the basic goals of treatment in cystic fibrosis? Why is aggressive nutritional therapy a main part of the treatment?

3. Outline a day's food plan for Paul. Check the amount of protein and kcalories by calculating total food values in your food plan to ensure the extra amount that he needs.

4. Why does Paul require enzyme replacement and therapeutic dosages of multivitamins, including the B complex? Why does he need to have his vitamins in water-soluble form?

Situational Problem: Bill's Bout with the Hepatitis A Virus (HAV)

Bill is a college student who spent part of his summer vacation in Mexico. Shortly after he returned home, he began to feel ill. He had little energy, no appetite, and severe headaches. Nothing he ate seemed to agree with him. He felt nauseated, began to have diarrhea, and soon developed a fever. He began also to show evidence of jaundice.

Bill was hospitalized for diagnosis and treatment. His tests indicated that he had impaired liver function and an enlarged, tender liver and spleen. The diagnosis indicated that he was infected with the hepatitis A virus (HAV), a common form of infectious hepatitis spread by contaminated food or water.

Bill's hospital diet was high in protein, carbohydrates, kcalories, and moderate in fats. However, Bill had difficulty eating. He had no appetite, and food seemed to nauseate him even more.

1. What significant metabolic functions of the liver relate to his handling of carbohydrates?

2. What are the functions of the liver in fat metabolism?

3. What are the functions of the liver in protein metabolism?

4. What other nutrient-related functions does the liver have?

5. What is the relationship of these normal liver functions to the effects, of clinical symptoms, that Bill experienced in his bout with the hepatitis A virus?

6. Why does vigorous nutritional therapy in liver disease such as hepatitis present such a problem in planning a diet?

7. Outline a day's food plan for Bill. Calculate the amount of kcalories and protein to ensure he is getting an optimum intake.

8. What vitamins and minerals would be significant aspects of Bill's nutritional therapy? Why?

Current Nutrition Issues

Read carefully the section on nutritional aspects of diarrhea (*Essentials of Nutrition and Diet Therapy* ed 6, p 355; *Nutrition and Diet Therapy*, ed 7, p 573). Consider these inquiry questions:

1.　　Why is infant diarrhea in particular a potentially dangerous condition?

2.　　How would the body's normal large gastrointestinal circulation of water and electrolytes influence the problem of diarrhea?

3.　　Why must effective nutritional therapy be based on the type of diarrhea present?

4.　　Why would general malnutrition result from continuing diarrhea?

Chapter 20
DISEASES OF THE HEART, BLOOD VESSELS, AND LUNGS

Chapter Focus

Since cardiovascular disease is the leading cause of death in the United States, control of identified risk factors is important in prevention and treatment of diseases affecting the overall circulatory system. Several of these factors relate to our food habits and are associated with fats and sodium.

Summary-Review Quiz

Fill in the blanks below with the appropriate number and word(s) from the list following each section. Each numbered word or phrase is used; some may be used more than once. When you have completed all the sections, check your answers for each blank by the test key (Appendix, p 277). Correct any mistakes and then review the entire chapter summary.

1. Multiple _____ factors contribute to the development of heart disease. Personal factors include: (1) strong _____ of heart disease, (2) _____ (greater incidence in men), (3) _____ (approximate range of 30 to 55 years), (4) _____, which influences hypertension and increases the heart workload, and (5) a _____ personality. Behavior habit patterns are also involved: (1) heavy _____, (2) _____ of food with greater quantities of _____ and _____, and (3) little or no physical _____. Associated conditions include (1) _____, (2) elevated blood _____, and (3) _____.

1. sex	6. diabetes	11. exercise
2. fats	7. smoking	12. excess amounts
3. overweight	8. stress-absorbing	13. sugar
4. hypertension	9. cholesterol	14. age
5. family history	10. risk	

2. The underlying disease process is _____, which is characterized by _____ deposits in _____ linings. This fact should lead to a focus on _____ metabolism with attention paid specifically to: (1) the fat-related compound _____, (2) _____ fats in the diet, and (3) various _____, the major blood lipid transport compound. Several different types of _____ have been identified, according to the forms of _____ that are elevated and the clinical symptoms displayed.

3. Various fat-controlled diets modify the _____ and kind of food fat used or the amount of dietary _____. Usually the diet restricts _____ from

animal food sources and _____ .

4. _____ may be decreased in initial stages of care after a heart attach to provide cardiac rest. The diet's _____ may also be modified to _____ or soft food forms to avoid effort in chewing or eating.

1. cholesterol
2. blood lipids
3. lipoproteins
4. kcalories
5. atherosclerosis
6. liquid
7. amount
8. saturated fat
9. blood vessel
10. texture
11. saturated
12. fatty
13. fat
14. lipid disorders

5. In _____ heart failure, diet therapy is used to control the _____ . The weakened _____ cannot sustain an adequate _____; so fluid backs up and accumulates in the _____ . The main cause of this _____ is an imbalance in the _____ mechanism. Also the action of two basic hormones contributes to the problem (1) _____ from the adrenal gland and (2) _____ from the pituitary gland. Both these hormones are triggered in response to the reduced _____ and _____ involved in the illness. Diet therapy centers on _____ of _____ to help control the _____ .

1. capillary fluid shift
2. tissues
3. restriction
4. ADH
5. heart muscle
6. sodium
7. blood output
8. stress
9. aldosterone
10. congestive
11. edema
12. circulating blood pressure

6. _____ is a state of elevated blood pressure. It is present in about _____ of the population. It may be _____ with cause unknown, or it may be associated with some other basic disease process. Diet therapy is aimed at restriction of _____ , with adequate amounts of two other minerals, _____ and _____ . _____ is also indicated if the patient is obese, along with a good _____ program.

7. Education of the patient and family in any form of _____ should stress the need for _____ care. Also, careful _____ of processed foods is necessary to avoid excess _____ , _____ , sugar, and _____ . The focus should be on _____ with early attention to _____ , especially for those with a strong _____ of heart disease or _____ .

1. sodium
2. weight loss
3. prevention
4. hypertension
5. risk factors
6. continuing
7. label-reading
8. calcium
9. kcalories
10. 20%
11. potassium
12. family history
13. exercise
14. fats
15. heart disease
16. essential hypertension

Discussion Questions

1. What does the word *saturated* mean as applied to fats? What is the physical nature of the respective fats, depending on the degree of saturation? Diagram the resulting food fat spectrum.

2. What is a lipoprotein? What is an apoprotein? What is the significance of these two components in cardiovascular disease?

3. What are the types of lipid disorders? What diet therapy should be used with each?

4. What probable roles in treatment of heart disease seem indicated by continuing study of additional dietary factors such as dietary fiber and omega-3 fatty acids?

5. What does the term *cardiac edema* mean? Describe the physiologic action involved in the four causes of cardiac edema found in congestive heart failure.

6. What drug and diet treatment is used in congestive heart failure? Why is it effective?

7. What nutritional factors are involved in treatment of hypertension? Why?

8. Describe the condition of chronic obstructive pulmonary disease in respiratory failure. How does the progressive respiratory failure affect the normal exchange of oxygen and carbon dioxide in the lungs? What are the special changed nutrient proportions used in nutritional management? Why?

Self-Test Questions

<u>True-False</u>
     Circle the "T" if a statement is true and write a brief rationale for its accuracy. If it is false, circle the "F" and write the correct statement.

T F   1.   Cardiovascular disease occurs most widely in underdeveloped countries of the world.

T F   2.   Heart disease occurs more in men who are "work addicts," spending long hours under pressure with little sleep or exercise.

T F   3.   A lean man is more likely to have a heart attack than is an overweight man.

T F   4.   In the disease process, atherosclerosis, the fatty deposits in blood vessel linings are composed mainly of cholesterol.

T F   5.   Hypertension occurs more in Black populations.

T F   6.   A myocardial infarction, or "heart attack," results from the cutting off of blood supply to a part of the heart muscle (myocardium).

T F   7.   The problem of cardiovascular disease could be solved if cholesterol could be removed entirely from the body.

T F   8.   Cholesterol is a dietary essential because humans depend entirely on food sources for their necessary supply.

T F   9.   "Hyperlipidemia" refers to elevated blood levels of fats.

T F 10. Lipoproteins are the major transport form of lipids in the blood.

T F 11. Saturated fats are usually liquid in form.

T F 12. About two thirds of the total fat in the American diet is of animal origins and therefore mainly saturated.

T F 13. Egg yolk is a major food source of cholesterol, each one containing almost 300 mg, which is the approximate daily total amount of cholesterol allowed on a low-cholesterol diet.

T F 14. The basic therapeutic objective in treatment of acute cardiovascular disease is cardiac rest.

T F 15. Coconut oil is a polyunsaturated vegetable oil, used in low-saturated fat diets.

T F 16. In congestive heart failure the heart fails because its muscle works at a faster rate and pumps out the returning blood too rapidly.

T F 17. The capillary fluid shift mechanism is the main means of maintaining the normal flow of fluids throughout the body.

T F 18. Aldosterone is a sodium- and therefore water-conserving hormone meant to be lifesaving, but in congestive heart failure it only compounds the problem of edema.

T F 19. The taste for salt is instinctive in man, to ensure that he will get a sufficient supply.

T F 20. Sodium restriction is effective therapy in congestive heart failure and hypertension.

T F 21. Regular cheese may be used on a low-sodium diet.
T F 22. Essential hypertension can be cured by drugs and diet.

Multiple Choice

Circle the letter in front of the correct answer. Then check your answers by the test key (Appendix, p 278). Now compare all the possible answers for each item and write the following brief statements: (1) rationale for the correct answer and (2) why each one of the other responses is incorrect.

1. Lipoproteins are produced in the body in the:
    (1) intestinal wall
    (2) spleen and bone marrow
    (3) liver
    (4) heart muscle
    a. 2 and 4
    b. 1 and 3
    c. 1 and 2
    d. 3 and 4
2. Chylomicrons are:
    a. small packets of enzymes for fat digestion
    b. a type of fatty acid
    c. a type of lipoprotein formed from dietary fat
    d. fat-bile complex formed for fat absorption
3. A low-cholesterol diet would restrict which of the following foods?
    (1) shellfish
    (2) liver
    (3) eggs
    (4) skimmed milk
    a. 1 and 3
    b. 2 and 3
    c. 3 and 4
    d. 1 and 4
4. The edema in congestive heart failure is caused by:
    (1) an imbalance in the capillary fluid shift mechanism
    (2) the aldosterone mechanism
    (3) the ADH mechanism
    (4) increased free cell potassium
    a. 2 and 3
    b. 2 and 4
    c. all of these
    d. 1 and 2

5.	Helpful seasonings to use on a sodium-restricted diet include:
	(1)	lemon juice
	(2)	soy sauce
	(3)	herbs and spices
	(4)	seasoned salt
	(5)	garlic or celery salt
	(6)	MSG (Accent)
	a.	1 and 3
	b.	2 and 4
	c.	5 and 6
	d.	1, 3, and 6
6.	Which of the following foods may be used freely on a low-sodium diet?
	a.	fruits
	b.	milk
	c.	meat
	d.	spinach and carrots

Learning Activities

Situational Problem: The Patient with a Myocardial Infarction

Robert Lewis is a successful business executive. He works long hours and carries the major responsibility in his corporation. At his last physical checkup, the physician cautioned him to slow his pace. Already he was having some mild hypertension. His blood cholesterol was elevated and he was overweight. In his desk job he got little exercise and found himself smoking more under tension. Although his annual income was quite high, his financial pressures seemed only to increase; he had several children in college and was trying to maintain the expensive home in the suburbs, which his wife, Barbara, seemed to enjoy.

One day while commuting on the freeway, he experienced a pain in his chest and vague apprehension. When he arrived home, the pain persisted and became more severe. He broke out into a cold sweat and felt nauseated. He thought that it was only indigestion because of eating dinner too rapidly. However, when he became more ill, his wife called their physician, and Robert was admitted to the hospital for care.

After emergency care and tests, the physician placed him in the coronary care unit at the hospital. His test results showed elevated cholesterol, lipoproteins, prothrombin time, SGOT, and LDH, and white blood cell count. The electrocardiogram revealed an infarction of the posterior wall of the myocardium.

At first Robert had only a liquid diet. As he began to feel better and his condition stabilized, his diet was increased to 800-kcal soft diet with low saturated fat. By the end of the first week, it was increased again to 1200-kcal full diet, low saturated fat, with only 25% of the total kcalories from fat, and a P/S ratio of 1.1 to 1.

Robert gradually improved over the next few weeks and finally was able to go home. The physician discussed with him the need for care at home during the period of convalescence. He explained that Robert had an underlying lipid disorder and was to continue his weight loss with a modified fat and carbohydrate diet.

1. What factors can you identify in Robert's background and personal medical history that place him in a "high-risk category" for coronary disease?
2. Account for the initial symptoms of Robert's illness. What happens in a myocardial infarction?
3. Identify as many of the laboratory tests that the physician ordered as you can. Relate these tests to cell metabolism. Why would they be elevated in Robert's case?
4. Why did Robert receive only a liquid diet at first?
5. What is the reason for each of the modifications in Robert's first diet of solid food?
6. What occurs in the disease process atherosclerosis?
7. What relation, if any, does fat metabolism have to the disease?
8. When Robert's diet was changed, what was meant by "P/S ratio of 1.1 to 1"?
9. Outline a day's menu for Robert on his increased diet of 1200 kcalories.
10. What needs might Robert have when he goes home? What plan would you make for helping him to prepare to go home?
11. Name some community resources that you might use in helping Robert understand his illness and its care.

Situational Problem: The Patient with Congestive Heart Failure

Mr. and Mrs. Natakis, age 75 and 73 years, have lived for some years in a small walk-up flat in a large city. They have a small income, barely enough to meet expenses if they plan carefully, based entirely on their small social security checks. They have no hospitalization insurance and know little about Medicare enrollment. They have no relatives nearby. Their two married sons live in a distant city and have had little contact with their parents in recent years.

For some time Mr. Natakis has been almost incapacitated with arthritis. He has had increasing difficulty with walking and caring for himself. Mrs. Natakis has been in fairly good health, although she has had hypertension for some years. She is grateful for her health, since she is able to take care of Mr. Natakis as he grows older. They are members of a Greek Orthodox church within walking distance of their apartment, to which Mrs. Natakis goes frequently to services. A small grocery store was located in the neighborhood, but in the past year the owner has not been able to continue his business, and it has closed. The nearest large supermarket is quite a distance from their apartment. However, Mrs. Natakis has been managing on the city bus, buying a few things at a time so that she could carry them back to the apartment.

Lately, however, she has noticed some shortness of breath when she climbs the stairs back to the apartment or walks a few blocks to their neighborhood church. She attributes this to her moderately increased weight. She is a short woman, 5 feet tall, and weighs 150 pounds.

Mrs. Natakis' efforts to reduce her weight in the past have been difficult because she is fond of the favorite Greek foods to which she has been accustomed all her life.

Frequently the couple have the salty cheeses. One of their favorite dishes, for example, consists of layers of potato and vegetables with cheese and spices, covered with a flaky, thin pastry. Mrs. Natakis still makes loaves of delicious bread, which they both enjoy and which is such a large part of every meal.

Today, walking back the two blocks from their church, Mrs. Natakis noticed increased difficulty breathing. As she started to climb the steps to their apartment, she could scarcely lift one foot above the other. She sat down on one of the steps, rested for awhile, and then tried to walk some more. Finally, she reached the apartment, after resting several times on the stairway. Inside the apartment she had increasing difficulty getting her breath. A neighbor came by and recognized her distress. She called the county hospital because Mr. and Mrs. Natakis had no routine medical care or regular physician and arranged to have her taken to the hospital for treatment.

At the hospital Mrs. Natakis was taken to the emergency room for care. After the physician's initial examination, he instituted therapy to relieve her difficulty in breathing. His diagnosis was listed as congestive heart failure and atherosclerotic heart disease with hypertension. He began treatment with diuretics and sedatives. She was taken to a bed on the medical ward, where the physician began a drug to strengthen heart action. He asked that the head of her bed be elevated, and the following day she was started on a diet of 500 mg of sodium.

Mrs. Natakis spent a fairly restful night, although she was having some difficulty. Her breathing, as well as her color, had improved the next morning when the physician checked with her again. He noted her response and changed the diet to 1200 kcal and 500 mg of sodium. Mrs. Natakis ate poorly when the first meals were brought to her, since she had little appetite and felt nauseated. As the days went by, however, she responded increasingly to her treatment, so that by the end of the first week the physician increased her dietary sodium limit to 1000 mg. After the second week the physician thought that she had improved sufficiently to leave the hospital. She was to continue carefully on the medications and the 1200-kcal, 1000-mg sodium diet.

1. What is congestive heart failure? What causes it?
2. What was the basic objective of the plan of therapy for Mrs. Natakis? By what means was this achieved?
3. The diuretic drugs used in Mrs. Natakis' treatment resulted in a loss of potassium. What foods could the nurse recommend to Mrs. Natakis as good sources of potassium, to ensure adequate replacement?
4. What personal factors need to be considered in planning a diet for Mrs. Natakis? What are some of the characteristics of Greek food habits?
5. What is the common amount of sodium in an average adult diet? What are the major sources of this dietary sodium?
6. What levels of sodium restriction are outlined in the American Heart Association diets in common use in the United States? What are the characteristics of each of these levels of sodium restriction?
7. Do you think Mrs. Natakis would find difficulty in accepting her low-sodium diet? Why?
8. How do you think that her food can be made more tasty?

9. Outline a day's menu for Mrs. Natakis on her 1200-kcal, 1000-mg sodium diet.

10. What practical problems will face Mrs. Natakis in buying her food and getting it into her apartment after she returns home? What solutions can you suggest?

Individual Project: Community Resources in Coping with Heart Disease

Make a visit to the local office of the Heart Association. Discuss the activities of this organization in patient education. Is a nutrition counselor available at the office? What resource materials do you find? Make a collection of these resources and prepare an exhibit of the materials.

Individual or Small Group Project: Fat-and Sodium-Modified Food Products

Visit several of your local food markets and survey the special modified food products designed for use on sodium-restricted or fat-modified diets. Include such items as margarines, coffee whiteners, milks, special egg substitute products, shortenings, oils, cheeses, and other fat-modified products. Check for sodium- or salt-free products such as canned vegetables, tomato juice, catsup, low-sodium cheese, and salt-free bread and margarine.

Evaluate these products in terms of taste and cost. If possible, prepare a "market basket" of such products to use in teaching patients.

Individual or Small Group Project: The Experience of a Heart Attach

Interview the public health nutritionist in your public health department or a physician in the community concerning any support and education program for coronary patients, such as a coronary club or clinic discussion group. If possible, visit one of these group sessions and observe the nature of the questions and concerns expressed by the group members.

Discuss in class the comparative findings of various class members in these visits. Why is a heart attack such a profound experience for a person?

Current Nutrition Issues

Read carefully the *Issues and Answers* article, "Is Calcium a New Risk Factor in Hypertension Control?" (*Essentials of Nutrition and Diet Therapy*, ed 6, p 412); *Nutrition and Diet Therapy*, ed 7, p 634). Consider these inquiry questions:

1. What are the claims being made by some researchers for the role of calcium in hypertension? What is the basis of these claims?

2. What are the five problems listed for the calcium-hypertension connections claimed by its proponents? Do these problems seem valid as indicated?

3.   How are calcium and sodium related in some food sources?

4.   What do newer current studies indicate concerning the role of sodium in hypertension? What is the recommendation of the American Heart Association and other health organizations?

Chapter 21
DIABETES MELLITUS

Chapter Focus

Sound nutritional therapy remains the fundamental base of management for all persons with diabetes. Wise food habits, together with newer insulins and self-monitoring of blood glucose, have become indispensable tools of good control and self-care.

Summary-Review Quiz

Fill in the blanks below with the appropriate number and word(s) from the list following each section. Each numbered word or phrase is used; some may be used more than once. When you have completed all the sections, check your answers for each blank by the test key (Appendix, p 278). Correct any mistakes and then review the entire chapter summary.

1. The underlying metabolic problem in diabetes is even yet _____. It is now evident that it is a condition with _____ forms, resulting from a _____ as in IDDM, or from _____ as in NIDDM. The hormone, _____, necessary for energy metabolism of the fuels _____, is not produced in sufficient _____ or _____ in the _____ by its special secretory cell clusters, the _____, to accomplish its designated metabolic job. Diabetes, in any event, then results from a _____, either at the _____ level in the _____ or at the _____ level in the blood.

2. Factors that predispose a person to the disease are (1) _____, a stronger factor in _____, which usually occurs in childhood and is _____ and unstable and (2) the metabolic stress of _____, a stronger factor in _____. The majority of persons with diabetes have a _____ form, _____, and are _____.

1. glucose and fat	8. genetic influences	15. obesity
2. production	9. quantity	16. unsolved
3. multiple	10. islets of Langerhans	17. pancreas islet cells
4. IDDM	11. availability	18. lack of insulin
5. form	12. insulin resistance	19. NIDDM
6. overweight	13. maturity onset	20. insulin-dependent
7. insulin	14. pancreas	

3. The initial symptoms of diabetes include excessive _____, urination, and hunger. Usually there is _____ with IDDM, depending on degree of disease process, and _____ with NIDDM. Further laboratory tests reveal: (1)

_____ in the urine—_____, (2) elevated _____ level—_____, and (3) abnormal _____ and _____ tests. In addition, individuals may complain of (1) _____ vision, (2) _____, and (3) infections. If the condition continues untreated, _____ from fluid and electrolyte imbalance and _____ from acid-base imbalance will follow. If untreated, eventually the patient will fall into a _____.

1. sugar	6. weight loss	11. thirst
2. skin irritation	7. ketoacidosis	12. blurred
3. 2-hour pc	8. fasting blood sugar	13. blood sugar
4. hyperglycemia	9. glycosuria	14. overweight
5. coma	10. dehydration	

4.   To maintain a proper _____ level, between _____ in the fasting state, the body must have (1) sources of _____, the diet and stored _____ and (2) ways of using _____, burning it for _____ or _____ it as _____ or _____ for future use. The hormone _____ controls these uses of _____. Hence it is a necessary agent for maintaining _____ balance. Another hormone also produced by the _____ has an opposite action to insulin and serves as a _____ hormone. This second hormone is _____. It helps to prevent _____ during fasting periods such as sleep hours.

1. glycogen	5. counterbalancing	9. blood glucose
2. fat	6. glucose	10. insulin
3. 70-120 mg/dl (4-6 mmol/L)	7. storing	11. pancreas
4. hypoglycemia	8. glucagon	12. energy

5.   The objectives of nutritional care in diabetes are: (1) optimum _____ with maintenance of ideal weight, (2) avoidance of _____ such as glycosuria and hyperglycemia, and (3) avoidance of _____ such as tissue changes in the _____, which affect vision, and in the nerves and _____.

6.   Basic control of diabetes rests on a balance of three important interrelated factors: (1) _____, the energy input source; (2) _____, the control agent; and (3) _____, the energy output use. Thus the fundamental concept of diabetes control is that of _____ (1) the overall _____ required to maintain ideal weight; (2) the _____ in foods consumed; more _____, _____, and moderate protein; and (3) the _____ of these foods throughout the day to match _____ and exercise. This control may be achieved by _____ in mild diabetes, by _____ in more involved cases, or by _____ in cases requiring greater control. In all cases a well-balanced, consistent _____ is the keystone of treatment.

1. eyes	7. symptoms	13. distribution balance
2. exercise	8. insulin activity	14. nutrition
3. complex carbohydrates	9. diet	15. diet and oral drugs
4. diet alone	10. energy balance	16. kidneys
5. balance	11. insulin	17. nutrient balance
6. diet and insulin	12. limited fat	18. complications

7.   To provide a flexible means of _____, the _____ system is a common tool. In this system, foods commonly used are grouped according to _____ and _____ value. These lists are called _____ groups. Then, within any one group, in the given _____, foods may be _____. A _____ using this system is worked out _____, and family as needed, which they may then use for planning _____. This basic system is a tool for providing both _____ and needed control.

1. energy	5. food variety	8. meal pattern
2. freely exchanged	6. like nutrient composition	9. diet planning
3. food exchange	7. daily menus	10. portion
4. with the patient		

8.   Throughout, the diet for any person with diabetes is always based on individual _____. Since control is largely in the _____, the key to successful management of diabetes lies in sound, realistic _____. Such a _____ program should include knowledge of (1) the _____; (2) all modes of managing diabetes, including _____; (3) methods of self-monitoring the disease status, including _____; (4) relation of _____ and skin care to good control; (5) _____ situations of insulin shock and acidosis, their prevention and treatment; (6) _____ and how to avoid them; (7) personal _____ in situations of need; (8) educational resources; and (9) _____ services and organizations.

1. disease process	5. community	9. identification
2. exercise	6. blood and urine testing	10. normal nutritional needs
3. patient's hands	7. patient education	11. emergency
4. complications	8. diet and drug therapy	12. diabetes education

Discussion Questions

1.   How do IDDM and NIIDM differ?

2.   Family history is a strong factor in diabetes. How are such diseases as diabetes inherited? What is a genetic disease? What is the "thrifty gene" hypothesis of diabetes development?

3.   Why are the islets of Langerhans called *endocrine glands within an exocrine gland?* How do these special cell clusters control the body's blood glucose balance? What hormones do these cell clusters produce and how do they interact?

4.   What are the current dietary recommendations for diabetes management concerning nutrient ratio and type (carbohydrate, fat, protein)? What possible role may dietary fiber play?

Self-Test Questions

<u>True-False</u>
        Circle the "T" if a statement is true and write a brief rationale for its accuracy. If it is false, circle the "F" and write the correct statement.

T F   1.   The majority of persons with NIDDM are underweight at the time the disease is discovered.

T F   2.   In females developing diabetes a common symptom that leads them to seek medical care, and discover the disease, is skin irritation of the vulva because of the heavy glucose load in the urine.

T F   3.   The two nutrients whose metabolism is most closely affected in diabetes are fat and protein.

T F   4.   Insulin is a hormone produced by the pituitary gland.

T F   5.   Insulin action is influenced by both glucagon and somatostatin.

T F   6.   Acetone in the urine of a person with diabetes usually indicates that the diabetes is in poor control.

T F   7.   Persons with diabetes can test their own blood glucose and regulate insulin, food and exercise accordingly.

T F   8.   Coronary artery disease occurs in persons with diabetes at about four times the rate in the general population.

T F   9.   A diabetic diet is a combination of specific foods that should remain constant.

T F   10.   Persons with unstable IDDM disease should follow a low-carbohydrate diet.

T F 11.   NPH is a short-acting insulin, covering only a 4- to 6- hour period.

Multiple Choice

        Circle the letter in front of the correct answer. Then check your answers by the test key (Appendix, p 279). Now compare all the possible answers for each item and write the following brief statements: (1) rationale for the correct answer and (2) why each one of the other responses is incorrect.

1.   Which of the following statements correctly describe the action of insulin?
        (1)   It controls the entry of glucose into the cells.
        (2)   It regulates the conversion of glucose to glycogen for storage in the liver and muscle.
        (3)   It stimulates the conversion of glucose to fat for storage as adipose fat tissue.
        (4)   It allows fat to be converted to glucose as needed to return the blood glucose levels to normal.
        a.   2, 3, and 4
        b.   1, 3, and 4
        c.   1, 2, and 3
        d.   1, 2, and 4

2.   Which of the following metabolic changes occur in uncontrolled diabetes?
        (1)   Blood glucose cannot enter the cell to furnish energy so it builds up in the blood.
        (2)   Fat formation is increased, and fat breakdown is decreased.
        (3)   Ketones from fat breakdown accumulate in the blood and appear in the urine.
        (4)   Tissue protein synthesis increases and urinary protein metabolites decrease.
        a.   1 and 2
        b.   3 and 4
        c.   2 and 4
        d.   1 and 3

3.   The caloric value of a diabetic diet should be:
        a.   increased above normal requirements to meet the increased metabolic demand
        b.   decreased below normal requirements to prevent glucose formation
        c.   the individual's normal energy requirement to maintain ideal weight
        d.   contributed mainly by fat to spare carbohydrate

4. In the exchange system of diet control an ounce of cheese equals:
    (1) the same amount of meat
    (2) one cup of milk
    (3) two tablespoons of peanut butter
    (4) 1/2 cup ice milk
    a. 1 and 3
    b. 2 and 4
    c. 1 and 4
    d. 2 and 3
5. The exchange system of diet control is based on principles of:
    (1) equivalent food values
    (2) variety of food choices
    (3) nutritional balance
    (4) reeducation of eating habits
    a. 1 and 3
    b. 2 and 4
    c. 2 and 3
    d. all of these

Learning Activities

Situational Problem: Jimmy and His Family Learn to Live with Diabetes

Jimmy, age 7, lives with his parents and two older brothers, ages 12 and 14. Recently he has begun to lose some of his usual energy. His mother also noticed that his weight was dropping steadily, despite the fact that he seemed hungry all the time and was eating a great deal. He was also drinking more water than usual and urinating more frequently. One morning when Jimmy felt too ill to go to school, his mother decided to take him to a physician. At the office the physician examined him carefully, talked with his mother, and did some simple urine and blood tests. As he had suspected, he found sugar in the urine and an elevated level in the blood.

When he told Jimmy's mother about his findings, he asked if there had been a family history of diabetes. She answered that she was not surprised because she had suspected this all along. "Jimmy's father has diabetes," she answered. "I guess we just didn't want to face the fact that Jimmy had diabetes because we knew we had given it to him."

The physician made arrangements for Jimmy to have some more definite tests so that his diabetes could be regulated. He also wanted all the family to have a careful plan of teaching.

Jimmy's diet therapy was started at 1600 kcal. The diet would need to be built up gradually as his diabetes became more regulated and he needed more food. The clinical dietitian indicated that the kcalories would be gradually increased to a maintenance level of about 2200 kcal for the present. Jimmy was to have three meals each day with snacks between meals and in the evening. He was receiving 15 units of NPH insulin, plus 5 units of regular insulin. Gradually his urine test, although still somewhat erratic, showed improvement.

Jimmy's nurse and clinical dietitian made plans for the necessary teaching. They talked with Jimmy's mother in great detail about the family's food habits and with other members of the health team who had occasion to observe Jimmy and his reaction to food in the hospital. They also contacted the nurse at Jimmy's school and reviewed his situation with her. Together they arranged for Jimmy to have the care he needed in any emergency that might arise.

1. What were the reasons for the initial symptoms that Jimmy experienced at home?
2. What implications for counseling might exist because of the hereditary nature of the disease?
3. If Jimmy's mother had not been alert and taken him to the physician when she did, what progression of his symptoms might have occurred? Account for these progressive symptoms by the chain of metabolic imbalances occurring in uncontrolled diabetes.
4. In planning the overall educational program for Jimmy and his parents, his nurse listed all the items important for a person with diabetes to know. What would she have included in her list? Why?
5. Outline a day's diet pattern and a sample food plan for Jimmy to use at home after he returns to school on a 2200 kcal diet. He is to continue with three meals and three snacks.
6. Why must Jimmy's insulin be given by hypodermic injection, rather than be taken as an oral mediation?
7. What is the relationship of the distribution of food throughout the day to balance with insulin activity and exercise? How would you explain this balance to Jimmy's mother?
8. What teaching materials or community resources could you use in an educational plan for Jimmy and his family?

Individual Project: Interviewing a Person with Diabetes

Have various members of the class interview persons with diabetes. Include both children and adults in the survey. Plan questions concerning the following items:

1. The person's feelings when he first learned that he first had diabetes
2. His experience with the disease—any emergencies, complications, or hospitalizations
3. If he has traveled, how he has managed his disease away from home
4. His regular method of management at home, school, or work, as well as social events
5. The kind of diet that he follows (If possible, to learn more about his diet, take a diet history according to the guidelines that you have learned in previous chapters. Evaluate your findings in terms of total energy intake in relation to his weight and general balance and nutrients.)

Have a class discussion after the interviews to compare the nature of diabetes and its management in the various persons that were contacted.

<u>Group Project: Community Diabetes Resources</u>

Explore any available community resources for diabetes. Investigate your local county or district chapter of the American Diabetes Association. Make an appointment with the local office director concerning the group's activities in patient education and other activities. If possible, visit a group meeting of the chapter members.

Also contact the nutritionist in your local country public health department to inquire about community resources for people with diabetes.

Current Nutrition Issues

Read carefully the *Issues and Answers* article "Questions from Persons on Diabetic Diets" (*Essentials of Nutrition and Diet Therapy*, ed 6, p 431; *Nutrition and Diet Therapy*, ed 7, p 659). Consider these inquiry questions:

1.   What negative effects does alcohol have for the person with diabetes?

2.   Are there any positive metabolic effects of alcohol in relation to diabetes?

3.   What specific instructions would a person with diabetes who chooses to drink need to control alcohol's effects on diabetes control?

4.   What advice would you give to your diabetic client about the use of alcohol? Why?

5.   How does fructose differ from sugar? How would you advise a person with diabetes about the use of fructose as a sweetener?

Chapter 22
RENAL DISEASE

Chapter Focus

Renal disease places great physical, personal, and financial burdens on the lives of many people, especially those with chronic failure who face daily dialysis treatment. Nutritional support therapy seeks to maintain optimal nutritional status and control carefully all affected nutrients in each person.

Summary-Review Quiz

Fill in the blanks below with the appropriate number and word(s) from the list following each section. Each numbered word or phrase is used; some may be used more than once. When you have completed all the sections, check your answers for each blank by the test key (Appendix p 280). Correct any mistakes and then review the entire chapter summary.

1. The work of the kidney is carried out by its many small functional units, the _____. This work consists of _____ the entering blood, _____ needed blood materials through the walls of the winding tubules, _____ additional ions as needed to maintain _____, and _____ unneeded materials in a concentrated urine.

2. Specific structures that accomplish these vital tasks are _____ at the head of the nephron for _____ the blood and winding tube of four successive sections:_____, _____, _____, and _____, for _____ materials, _____ ions, _____ the urine, and _____ unneeded materials in it.

1. secreting	5. concentrating	9. acid-base balance
2. excreting	6. nephrons	10. distal tubule
3. loop of Henle	7. reabsorbing	11. glomeruli
4. collecting tubule	8. proximal tubule	12. filtering

3. Various diseases of the kidney interfere with these normal functions. A previous streptococcal infection may lead to acute _____, in which the disease process causes loss of the normal _____ function of _____. In short-term acute cases in children a diet _____ in protein or sodium from the child's normal diet.

4. In cases of _____ the basement membrane of the _____ degenerates and develops large "pores." This permits large amounts of _____, mainly in the form of _____, to be lost in the urine. With loss of _____, the _____ mechanism begins to fail. Fatty tissue changes

develop in the _____, and general _____ follows. All these events cause severe _____, especially in the abdomen and legs. Diet therapy centers on _____ replacement, with a diet moderate in _____ and further individual _____ only according to daily urinary loss. Sufficient _____ are provided to ensure _____ use for tissue synthesis. Restriction of _____ helps combat the severe edema.

1. nephrotic syndrome
2. capillary fluid shift
3. glomerulonephritis
4. albumin
5. kcalories
6. filtering
7. sodium
8. glomeruli
9. fluid accumulation
10. glomerular
11. liver
12. is not modified
13. malnutrition
14. protein
15. protein supplement

5.   Progressive degeneration of renal tissue leads to _____. Treatment is highly individual, depending on the patient's specific degree of _____ remaining. The general objective is to correct the specific _____ created by the degree of disease involvement, especially to control _____, _____, and _____ balances. Depending on degree of function, the predialysis diet for advanced disease restricts _____ to _____ a day and uses only _____, either in foods or special _____, thus causing the body to use its own excess urea nitrogen to synthesize the _____ needed for tissue protein production. The general routine used for most dialysis patients is more _____ with normal amounts of _____. Treatment centers on maintaining _____ and relieving the severe _____.

1. protein
2. formulas
3. nitrogen imbalance
4. essential amino acids
5. water
6. protein and kcalories
7. kidney function
8. 20 to 25 g
9. clinical symptoms
10. liberal
11. chronic renal failure
12. optimal nutrient balances
13. nonessential amino acids
14. electrolyte

6.   Kidney stones varying in _____ may form from a number of contributing factors, relating to the nature of the _____ or to the condition of the _____ environment. According to their main chemical composition, these kidney stones may be of four types: (1) _____, by far the most prevalent; (2) _____ stones, often associated with urinary tract infections; (3) _____, from increased breakdown of protein, especially _____ as in gout; and (4) _____, from a _____ defect in handling its precursor, essential amino acid _____. A basic objective of diet therapy for the three dietary nutrient-related stones mentioned is to reduce the intake of the stone constituent involved: (a) _____ with additional restriction of the _____ in the stone compound, (b) _____, and (c) _____.

7.   In addition, the diet may be modified according to its influence on urinary acidity. This diet may be designed to create an _____ to treat cases of the most prevalent

stone or an _____ to treat cases of the less common ones.

1. calcium compounds
2. low methionine diet
3. calcium partner
4. uric acid
5. low purine diet
6. urine
7. alkaline ash
8. urinary tract
9. cystine
10. low calcium diet
11. acid ash
12. size and chemistry
13. methionine
14. struvite magnesium
15. genetic
16. purines

Discussion Questions

1. What causes the massive edema seen in nephrotic syndrome? Account for this major problem by describing the various malfunctions that combine to produce it.

2. How are individual patients with nephrotic syndrome currently being treated to achieve better metabolic balance? Describe this new diet therapy and give its rationale.

3. What nutrients need close monitoring in predialysis chronic renal failure? How are these nutrients modified in the patient's diet? Give reasons for each modification as you would explain them to a patient.

4. Why is the diet for a dialysis patient more liberal? Why do you think that this liberal diet transition may be difficult for a dialysis patient to make?

5. Can an acid ash diet dissolve an already formed calcium kidney stone? Why or why not? What is the diet's effect?

Self-Test Questions

<u>True-False</u>

Circle the "T" if a statement is true and write a brief rationale for its accuracy. If it is false, circle the "F" and write the correct statement.

T F 1. The basic functional unit of the kidney is the nephron.

T F 2. There are only a few nephrons in each kidney; so a metabolic stress load can easily cause problems.

T F 3. The operation of the nephrons has little relation to the rest of the body.

T F 4. The task of the glomerulus is filtration.

T F 5. At the glomerulus all the blood constituents are normally filtered through, except for the blood cells and the plasma protein.

T F 6. Most of the major nutrient substances in the filtrate are then reabsorbed back into the blood in the final section of the nephron tubule.

T F 7. By the time the filtrate reaches the midsection of the nephron tubule, the loop of Henle, about 70% to 85% of it has already been reabsorbed.

T F 8. In the latter portion of the tubule, aldosterone acts to cause reabsorption of sodium.

T F 9. In the final collecting section of the tubule, ADH acts to cause reabsorption of water and thus help dilute the urine.

T F 10. The urine is concentrated by the loop of Henle's work in increasing the density of the fluid surrounding the nephron.

T F 11. The resulting volume of urine ready for excretion is only 0.5% to 1% of the volume of the original filtrate formed at the glomerulus.

T F 12. Diet modifications in acute glomerulonephritis usually involve crucial restrictions of protein and sodium.

T F 13. The primary symptom in nephrotic syndrome is massive albuminuria.

T F 14. Chronic renal failure occurs in advanced renal insufficiency.

T F 15. The multiple symptoms of advanced chronic renal failure result from the elevated blood urea levels.

T F 16. A special high-protein bread is used in the diet for chronic renal failure.

T F 17. Prolonged immobilization, as in body casting or long-term illness or disability, may lead to withdrawal of bone calcium and the formation of calcium renal stones.

T F 18. Cystine stones, caused by a rare hereditary metabolic defect in renal tubular reabsorption of cystine, are treated by direct dietary control of the amino acid cystine.

T F 19. Persons living in a dry, hot climate, as in the desert, are more prone to develop kidney stones.

Circle the letter in front of the correct answer. Then check your answers by the test key (Appendix, p 281). Now compare all the possible answers for each item and write the following brief statements: (1) rationale for the correct answer and (2) why each one of the other responses is incorrect.

1. Acute glomerulonephritis is best treated by:
   (1) reducing protein, since filtration is impaired
   (2) leaving protein at normal levels for optimum tissue nutrition
   (3) restricting sodium to help control edema
   (4) allowing salt in the diet in uncomplicated acute cases
   a. 1 and 3
   b. 2 and 4
   c. 1 and 2
   d. 3 and 4

2. Symptoms of nephrotic syndrome revealed by blood and urine test may include:
   (1) large urinary loss of albumin
   (2) urinary loss of special thyroid-binding protein
   (3) urinary loss of special iron-binding protein
   (4) a rise in serum cholesterol levels as blood levels of plasma protein drop
   a. 1 and 3
   b. 1 and 4
   c. all of these
   d. 1 and 2

3. The loss of protein in nephrotic syndrome leads to:
   (1) fatty infiltration of the liver because of lack of adequate protein
   (2) gross edema because of loss of sufficient plasma protein
   (3) increased breakdown of tissue protein
   (4) general overall malnutrition and weight loss
   a. 2 and 3
   b. 1 and 4
   c. 2 and 4
   d. all of these

4. Current diet therapy in nephrotic syndrome is designed to:
   (1) use a high-protein diet to replace the massive losses
   (2) moderately restrict regular dietary protein to protect nephrons and add protein supplement according to individual urinary loss
   (3) increase kcalories to provide energy and ensure protein for needed tissue synthesis
   (4) decrease kcalories to reduce metabolic work load
   (5) restrict sodium to combat the massive edema
   (6) use only mild sodium restriction, to aid food taste and assure optimum food intake
   a. 2, 3, and 5
   b. 1, 4, and 6
   c. 1, 4, and 5
   d. 2, 3, and 6

5. The symptoms of chronic renal failure usually include:
   (1) anemia
   (2) weight loss
   (3) high blood pressure
   (4) weakness
   (5) bone and joint pain
   a. all of these
   b. 1, 2, and 3
   c. 1, 2, and 4
   d. 2, 3, and 4

6. The treatment objectives in chronic renal failure include:
   (1) reduction of protein breakdown
   (2) control of water and electrolyte balance
   (3) maintenance of nutrition and weight by supporting appetite and morale
   (4) control of acid-base balance
   (5) control of complications of hypertension, bone pain, and central nervous system abnormalities
   a. 1, 2, and 3
   b. 3, 4, and 5
   c. 2, 3, and 4
   d. all of these

7. The general diet needs in chronic renal failure include:
   (1) reduced protein intake
   (2) increased carbohydrate and fat, as needed for energy and protein sparing
   (3) careful control of sodium and potassium, according to individual need
   (4) increased fluid intake to stimulate kidney function
   a. 1, 2, and 3
   b. 2, 3, and 4
   c. 1, 3, and 4
   d. 1, 2, and 4

8. The diet therapy indicated for a patient with calcium phosphate kidney stones would be:
   a. low calcium and phosphorus, alkaline ash
   b. high calcium and phosphorus, acid ash
   c. low calcium and phosphorus, acid ash
   d. high calcium and phosphorus, alkaline ash
9. The diet therapy indicated for a patient with cystine stones would be:
   a. low methionine, alkaline ash
   b. low purine, alkaline ash
   c. low protein, acid ash
   d. low calcium, acid ash
10. Which of the following foods would be restricted on a low-purine diet for uric acid stones?
    (1) liver
    (2) meat broth or gravy
    (3) eggs
    (4) milk
    a. 1 and 3
    b. 2 and 4
    c. 1 and 2
    d. 3 and 4
11. In planning a diet for patient with calcium phosphate kidney stones, which of the following foods could you use in liberal amounts?
    a. fruits
    b. meat
    c. milk
    d. cheese

Learning Activities

Situational Problem: The Patient with Chronic Renal Failure

David Parker, age 45, is an active, energetic man employed by a large company. His wife, Mary, works as an administrative assistant for a business executive. They have three healthy, vigorous children, a boy 18, and two girls, 16 and 14. They are a close, busy family.

Over a period of time, David has begun to tire more easily. He has no appetite and feels nauseated and ill a great part of the time. Recently, he began to notice some ankle swelling and blood in his urine. Finally, at Mary's insistence he decided to see his physician.

The physician gave David a thorough examination. He learned that David had suffered a rather severe case of influenza accompanied by throat infection during an epidemic in his company when he was overseas in the army. David said that no other major illnesses had occurred and that he had been well until these symptoms started. The physician had a number of laboratory tests done, and he asked David to return in about 2 weeks or sooner if his symptoms changed. When the laboratory test results returned, they showed albumin, red and white cells in the urine, and elevated BUN and GFR. The urine showed a high specific gravity. Other symptoms included hypertension, edema, headache, occasional vision blurring, and a low-grade fever.

When David returned to see the physician, these findings were discussed. They indicated chronic renal failure, probably the result of the previous infectious illness. The physician discussed with David the serious prognosis of the disease process, and together they explored the alternatives of medical management with kidney dialysis when needed and kidney transplant surgery. He began David's medications to control the hypertension and to ease his growing discomforts and symptoms.

As time went by, David's symptoms increased. He lost more weight, was anemic, and was having increased aching in his bones and joints. He had to conduct numerous public meetings in which he made speeches, but he reached the point when he could not stand at these conferences and would sit as often as he could. Gastrointestinal bleeding and nausea also increased, with occasional muscular twitching or spasms. Numerous small mouth ulcers made eating a painful effort. David and Mary discussed candidly the prospects before them. They decided that they would prefer to have the kidney transplant surgery that the physician had suggested as a possible therapy.

The nutritionist and the nurse arranged several clinic appointments for Mary so that she could learn how to care for David at home. The nutritionist outlined a definite meal pattern with food selection lists to provide precise control of protein, sodium, and potassium. She gave Mary many practical suggestions for obtaining and preparing the foods that David needed. David and Mary also learned how to use continuous ambulatory peritoneal dialysis (CAPD) while awaiting the kidney transplant surgery.

1. What metabolic imbalances in chronic renal failure do you think accounted for the characteristic symptoms that David displayed?
2. What are the objectives of treatment in chronic renal failure?
3. What would be the basic principles of David's predialysis nutritional therapy? Describe this type of diet. What foods would be included? How would the diet be planned?
4. What nutrient-related medications and supplements would David's physician and clinical nutritionist probably use in his treatment plan? Why?
5. Describe the process of CAPD.

Situation Problem: The Patient with Kidney Stones

Jim Roberts, age 25, lives in a small walk-up studio apartment in Manhattan, where he teaches school with a group of other young teachers in a hardcore urban ghetto community. He has group medical coverage through his employment in the city school system. He has been well during the past year except for several bouts with a recurring urinary tract infection. On one occasion he had suffered some renal colic and passed several small stones.

Jim eats sporadically, getting little for breakfast before he leaves the apartment, having a sandwich for lunch at school and eating irregularly in the evening at dinner time. Sometimes he gets involved in reading or studying and skips dinner altogether, getting snacks through the evening and drinking several glasses of milk. Occasionally he has dinner at a small neighborhood restaurant near his apartment. He drinks a great deal of milk, a carry-over habit from his childhood. His mother had always told him that is was "a perfect food," and besides, it was easy to keep and filling. Most days he drinks about two quarts at least. He is also fond of ice cream and could eat as much as a quart at a time.

During the past month or so, Jim has been feeling increasing pain through his right flank and back. He mentioned this to Susan, his girl friend, who encouraged him to see a physician. However, since the pain passed, he put off checking into it. One day, however, the pain became so severe that he could not go to school. He telephoned the principal to report his illness. He began to have chills. When he took his temperature, it was 100° F.

When Susan came by Jim's apartment after school to see how he was, she found him nauseous, vomiting, and in severe pain. She called his physician and drove him immediately to the hospital. After the hospital examination the physician decided to keep Jim in the hospital for several days for studies to determine what treatment would be needed. The results of the studies indicated normal kidney function and normal uric acid levels. However, there was some elevation of urinary calcium and serum calcium and phosphorus. X-rays indicated the presence of a rather large stone in the kidney pelvis on the left side. The physician ordered a diet for Jim of 400 mg of calcium and 1000 mg of phosphorus, acid ash. He also asked the nurse to force fluids.

As Jim's pain diminished and he began to feel better, the physician had him walk around the ward as much as possible. After a few more days of observation, the decision was made to remove the kidney stone surgically. Jim tolerated the surgery well, and his recovery was rapid.

1. What conditions predispose a person to the formation of kidney stones? Which of these factors may have been operative in Jim's case?
2. What do the results of the tests indicate that the probable chemistry of Jim's kidney stone was? What kind of stone do the test results rule out?
3. What are the reasons for Jim's specific diet therapy?
4. Outline a day's menu for Jim on his special diet. Calculate the amount of calcium and phosphorus to ensure control of each factor.
5. When Jim was ready to go home and needed instructions concerning his diet, what suggestions would you have given him? What problems would he face in carrying it out? What solutions would you propose?
6. What does "urinary ash" mean? What foods produce an alkaline ash? What foods produce an acid ash? What is the value of such a dietary modification in case of renal calculi or urniary tract infections?

Individual or Group Project: Kidney Dialysis Center

Assign individuals in the class to visit a kidney dialysis center if one is near enough to your community. Observe the operation of the center and discuss the diet used with the patients. If any teaching materials or diet guides are available, bring them back to the class for use in reporting your visit.

Current Nutritional Issues

Read carefully the *Issues and Answers* article "Technology vs. the Quality of Life" (*Essentials of Nutrition and Diet Therapy*, ed 6, p 452; *Nutrition and Diet Therapy*, ed 7, p 682). Consider these inquiry questions:

1.   What do you think are some of the ethical questions that may be increasingly involved in our rapidly advancing medical technology? Give examples.

2.   How do you view the quality of life balance with extended length of life?

3.   Why do you think many dialysis patients report that their lives are essentially as "normal" as usual?

4.   Do you know any persons on renal dialysis? What do you find their attitudes to be toward the quality of their lives? What alternatives do they have?

Chapter 23
NUTRITIONAL CARE OF SURGERY PATIENTS

Chapter Focus

Nutritional support is an essential component of therapy for all surgical patients to prevent catabolism, meet increased metabolic demands, avoid clinical problems, and promote wound healing and more rapid recovery. Various feeding modes, enteral and parenteral, may be used to meet postoperative nutritional goals according to individual needs.

Summary-Review Quiz

Fill in the blanks below with the appropriate number and word(s) from the list following each section. Each numbered word or phrase is used; some may be used more than once. When you have completed all the sections, check your answers for each blank by the test key (Appendix, p 282). Correct any mistakes and then review the entire chapter summary.

1.   Nutritional demands are greatly _____ by the physiologic stress of surgery. Nutrient _____ produce serious clinical problems.
2.   When time permits elective surgery, _____ nutritional preparation should correct nutrient _____ and provide nutrient _____ for the surgery and the _____ period. Special attention should be given to (1) building _____ reserves, (2) providing sufficient additional _____ kcalories for _____ and supporting optimum tissue stores, and (3) _____ for regulating _____ process.

1. preoperative	5. vitamins and minerals	9. energy
2. protein	6. postoperative	10. eficiencies
3. nonprotein	7. reserves	
4. increased	8. metabolic	

3.   Postoperative nutritional demands focus on the need for _____. Negative _____ is caused by losses in (1) _____ from tissue breakdown and infection and (2)_____ through would bleeding and exudate. Increased _____ is required to (1) supply the essential amino acids for _____, (2) avoid shock from reduced blood _____ resulting from loss of _____, (3) control _____ resulting also from lowered _____ osmotic pressure, thus helping to keep fluid circulating; (4) provide a sound matrix for _____; (5) build defense barriers, such as _____ against infection; and (6) provide carriers for fat transport in the blood as _____.

1. wound healing   5. nitrogen balance   9. protein
2. bone healing   6. edema   10. volume
3. antibodies   7. lipoproteins
4. tissue protein   8. plasma protein

4.   A vital concern after surgery is _____ to prevent dehydration. Large _____ may result from hemorrhaging, diuresis, vomiting, fever, and _____ of wounds or gastrointestinal suction. In complicated surgery with extensive drainage, as much as _____ of water may be required _____.

5.   Since increased _____ is needed for tissue synthesis, _____ must also be increased to supply energy demands and spare _____. In acute stress, as in extensive radical surgery or _____, as much as _____ kcal may be required.

6.   Increased amounts of _____ are needed for wound healing to provide the necessary _____ to build strong connective tissue. Additional _____ are needed as coenzyme control agents in energy production and tissue building. _____ is essential to proper blood clotting. Vitamin B_{12}, folic acid, and _____ are needed for hemoglobin formation.

1. daily   6. serious water losses   11. vitamin K
2. 7 liters   7. B vitamins   12. burns
3. 4000 to 6000   8. iron   13. water balance
4. protein   9. vitamin C   14. kcalories
5. cementing substance   10. tube drainage

7.   A return to _____ as soon as possible is desirable, but sometimes _____ methods may be required. In cases of _____ or gastrointestinal surgery, when a patient is unable to take sufficient nutrients for an extended period of time by _____ means, special vein feeding of _____ nutrient solutions may be needed to provide necessary _____.

8.   Nutritional care of patients with _____ surgery presents special needs. Surgery involving the mouth, throat, or neck requires a modified _____, either in oral liquid form with enriched drinks or in nutrient formulas fed by a _____. Usually one of the many _____ modified according to various clinical needs is used.

1. parenteral   6. alternate feeding methods
2. gastrointestinal   7. nutrition support
3. oral feeding   8. manner of feeding
4. commercial formulas   9. enteral
5. nasogastric or enterostomy tube   10. major tissue damage

9.   Stomach surgery requiring some degree of _____ requires a cautious resumption of oral feeding. Usually some form of surgical _____ meets

immediate postoperative needs. Initial oral meals should be _____ and frequent, and the type of food should be simple and easily digested. The _____ may be a later complication when greater _____ of concentrated foods are consumed and pass _____ into the upper intestine, causing shock symptoms from the _____ that follows. This reaction is avoided by using frequent _____ dry meals, low in concentrated _____ and high in _____ and fat.

10. A_____ procedure for surgical removal of the gallbladder requires some degree of _____ for a period of time, according to _____ needs.

1. fluid and electrolyte imbalance
2. simple carbohydrate
3. amounts and variety
4. gastrectomy
5. small
6. cholecystectomy
7. individual
8. protein
9. dumping syndrome
10. fat control
11. tube feeding
12. rapidly

11. After _____ surgery, resection and an 'ostomy procedure, some initial control of food _____ is required, but a return to a _____ as soon as tolerated is desirable. This provides optimum nutrients for healing and recovery and gives psychologic support to the patient. After rectal surgery, a _____ or _____ diet may be used briefly to delay initial bowel movements until healing has begun.

12. The patient with extensive _____ presents a crucial problem in nutritional care. After the immediate _____ period when oral feeding is resumed, rigorous _____ therapy with a diet high in _____, _____, and _____, with _____ as needed, is essential to initial _____. Follow-up skin _____ and plastic surgery continue this need for _____. Much continued _____ is needed to encourage eating and achieve nutritional goals.

1. residue-free
2. supplements
3. shock and recovery
4. grafting
5. protein
6. low-residue
7. nutritional support
8. healing
9. normal full diet
10. nutritional
11. personal support
12. texture
13. vitamins and minerals
14. burns
15. kcalories
16. intestinal

Discussion Questions

1.   Compare the nutrient and energy value of postoperative regular fluid-electrolyte intravenous feeding and oral feeding. Why is a rapid return to oral feeding important? What foods or drink could you use on a full liquid diet to supply extra needed protein and kcalories?

2.   What types of commercial formula preparations are available to supply increased nutrient and energy needs? In what kind of surgery cases would such feedings be required, fed by a nasoenteric tube?

3.   Why is vigorous nutritional therapy so crucial in caring for patients with extensive burns?

Self-Test Questions

True-False
        Circle the "T" if a statement is true and write a brief rationale for its accuracy. If it is false, circle the "F" and write the correct statement.

T F 1.   Usually nothing is given by mouth for at least 8 hours before surgery to avoid food aspiration during anesthesia.
T F 2.   The most common nutrient deficiency related to surgery is that of protein.
T F 3.   Negative nitrogen balance is a rare finding after surgery.
T F 4.   Extensive drainage in complicated surgery cases increases water loss to dangerous levels if constant replacement is not provided.
T F 5.   Vitamin D is essential to wound healing, since it provides a cementing substance to build strong connective tissue.
T F 6.   Oral liquid feedings usually provide little nourishment regardless of the type.
T F 7.   A postgastrectomy patient can usually return to regular eating within a few days.
T F 8.   The shock-producing postgastrectomy complex of symptoms is more precisely called the *jejunal hyperosmolic syndrome*.
T F 9.   After the diseased gallbladder is removed surgically, a postcholecystectomy patient can tolerate freely any food containing fats.
T F 10.   The management of an ileostomy and colostomy is the same.

T F 11. Commercial residue-free products provide a helpful means of feeding a patient after rectal surgery.

T F 12. A careful diet record of the total food and liquid intake is important for a burned patient to ensure that increased nutrient demands are met.

Multiple Choice

Circle the letter in front of the correct answer. Then check your answers by the test key (Appendix, p 283). Now compare all the possible answers for each item and write the following brief statements: (1) rationale for the correct answer and (2) why each one of the other responses is incorrect.

1. Postsurgical edema develops as a result of:
   a. decreased plasma protein levels
   b. excess water intake
   c. excess sodium intake
   d. lack of early ambulation and physical exercise
2. In the diet of a postoperative orthopedic patient, protein is essential to:
   a. provide extra energy needed to regain strength
   b. provide a matrix for anchoring mineral matter to form bone tissue
   c. control the basal metabolic rate
   d. give more satiety to the diet and thus increase appetite
3. Protein substances involved in the body defense mechanisms against infections include:
   (1) antigens
   (2) antibodies
   (3) blood cells
   (4) hormones
   (5) enzymes
   a. 1, 2, and 3
   b. 1, 2, and 5
   c. 2, 3, and 5
   d. 2, 3, 4, and 5
4. Complete dietary protein of high biologic value is essential to tissue building and wound healing after surgery because it:
   a. supplies all the essential amino acids needed for tissue synthesis
   b. spares carbohydrate to supply the necessary energy
   c. is easily digested and does not cause gastrointestinal upsets
   d. provides the most concentrated source of calories

5.　A diet for the dumping syndrome encountered by many patients after convalescence from a gastrectomy should include:

(1)　small frequent meals
(2)　no liquid with meals
(3)　no milk, sugar, sweets, or desserts
(4)　high-protein content
(5)　relatively high-fat content

a.　1, 4, and 5
b.　1, 2, and 3
c.　3, 4, and 5
d.　all of these

6.　A diet high in protein and kcalories is essential for a patient with extensive burns to:

(1)　replace the extensive tissue protein lost at the burn sites
(2)　provide essential amino acids for extensive tissue healing
(3)　counteract the negative nitrogen balance
(4)　meet added metabolic demands of infection or fever

a.　1 and 2
b.　1 and 4
c.　1 and 3
d.　all of these

Learning Activities

Situational Problem: The Patient with a Gastrectomy

After a long experience with peptic ulcer disease and little relief gained by conservative medical management, Charles Thompson and his physician decided that surgery would be the best treatment to follow. Charles then entered the hospital for a total gastrectomy.

The following day the surgeon performed the operation and established an anastomosis between the jejunum and the remaining portion of the esophagus. Charles withstood the surgery well and received some initial nutritional support from the elemental formula fed through a needle-catheter jejunostomy. Gradually, over the next 2-week period an oral refeeding program was initiated.

Since Charles tolerated initial fluids well, he was given the next few days a soft diet in small feedings about six times during the day. The nurse cautioned him to use his fluids, such as milk, soup, fruit juice, and other beverages, in moderation.

After Charles recovered from the surgery and was improved enough to go home, he gradually felt his strength returning. The clinical nutritionist had emphasized that he should observe his tolerances, eat small amounts at a time, and stress the use of protein foods. When Charles had recovered from the surgery itself and began to resume more and more of his usual activities, his food intake increased. Because he felt so much better, he began to eat a greater volume and variety of food. Friends invited the family out for meals, and they began to do entertaining themselves. Also he began to become involved more in his old business activities, in which many luncheon business conferences with rich foods and alcohol were included.

As time went by, Charles began experiencing increasing discomfort after his meals. About 10 to 15 minutes after he had eaten, he would have a cramping, full feeding. He felt his heart begin to beat more rapidly, and a wave of weakness would suddenly come over him. He would break out in a cold sweat and feel dizzy. Often he would become nauseated and vomit. As these episodes increased, his anxiety about himself increased accordingly, and as a result he started to eat less and less. His weight began to drop. He was already fairly thin, and this increased weight loss made him look more emaciated and debilitated. Soon he was in a general state of malnutrition.

When Charles returned to seek medical help, the physician and clinical nutritionist initiated a change in his eating habits. The clinic nurse described in general what the diet changes would be and made arrangements for both Charles and his wife to see the nutritionist, who then explained the diet in detail and worked out a food plan that would be acceptable in his situation. The diet seemed strange to Charles, but be began to follow it carefully. Because he felt so ill, he was glad to make any changes that might be helpful. To his pleased surprise he found that the symptoms he had experienced before disappeared almost completely. Because he felt so much better on the new diet plan, he formed his new eating habits around it. His weight gradually increased, and his general state of nutrition improved markedly. He found that he always fared better if he would nibble, rather than consume a large, heavy meal at one time.

1. What were Charles' nutritional needs immediately after surgery and in the next 2 weeks? Why was it necessary for his feedings to be resumed cautiously?
2. Why was an emphasis placed on protein intake after Charles' surgery, as he began to tolerate food? Why is a negative nitrogen balance a usual follow-up to surgical procedures? Why does the body need protein after surgery? What are its functions during this period?
3. Why do sufficient kcalories have to be consumed as soon as tolerated?
4. Why is fluid therapy of paramount importance after surgery?
5. What minerals and vitamins should be increased after surgery? Why?
6. When Charles began to feel better and resume heavier eating habits, why did he experience the symptoms he did after consuming a meal? What is this response called? Why?
7. What principles of diet therapy would have been followed in the corrective diet suggestions given to Charles by the physician, the nurse, and the nutritionist? Give reasons for each of these principles.
8. Outline a day's meal pattern for Charles on his newly adjusted diet pattern.

Individual or Group Project: Elemental Diets

Make a survey to discover as many as possible of the commercial products available for use as elemental diets. The name "elemental diet" is generally used to describe diets in which protein is present in predigested or elemental form as protein

216

hydrolysates or synthetic amino acids and carbohydrate and fat are present in simple, readily digestible form. Vitamins and minerals are present also to assure complete nutrition. Such preparations are almost totally absorbed in the upper intestine, leaving little residue to reach the large bowel. They are used frequently with surgical patients.

To gather information about these various products, interview a nutritionist or a surgeon who is involved in their use. Also survey available products in a community drugstore or discuss them with a pharmacist. Look for product advertisements in the *Journal of the American Dietetic Association*. Locate as many items as you can and compare these products as to nutrient composition and cost. Discuss your findings with others in the class who have also participated in the survey. What conclusions can you reach concerning the use of such products?

Current Nutrition Issues

Read carefully the *Issues and Answers* article, " New Methods of Assessing Nutritional Status?" (*Essentials of Nutrition and Diet Therapy*, ed 6, p 467, *Nutrition and Diet Therapy*, ed 7, p 699). Consider these inquiry questions:

1. Distinguish between *objective* and *subjective* nutritional assessment measures. Give examples of each type of measure.

2. What comparative value had you given to each of these two evaluation approaches before reading of this research with surgical patients using what the researchers called a "subjective global assessment"?

3. Has this study altered your thinking about relative values of these two types of nutritional status assessment? If so, in what way?

Chapter 24
NUTRITION AND AIDS

Chapter Focus

The current spread of the human immunodeficiency virus (HIV) and its deadly end stage of acquired immunodeficiency syndrome (AIDS) has become pandemic in the nations of the world. As knowledge of the disease process has grown over the past decade, it has become increasingly clear that in each of the distinct stages of the disease nutritional support plays a vital role in the care of HIV-infected and AIDS patients.

Summary-Review Quiz

Fill in the blanks below with the appropriate number and word(s) from the list following each section. Each numbered word or phrase is used; some may be used more than once. When you have completed all the sections, check your answers for each blank by the test key (Appendix, p 283). Correct any mistakes and then review the entire chapter summary.

1.   AIDS apparently first gained its hold in the central African country of _____ and its _____ effects have since spread worldwide. The infectious agent is now known to be a _____ and has been named _____ to distinguish it from another African strain _____. Both of these strains are genetically similar to a type found in African primates called _____ and were probably transmitted to human hunters in earlier ages, slowly evolving over time.

2.   Rapidly increasing _____ and _____ of the past few decades have greatly accelerated _____ transmission and multiplication. Its current deadly strength results from its _____ in an increasing number of _____.

3.   Today more than _____ people throughout the world are infected with _____, with the majority living in _____ where the first cases appeared. However, increased urbanization in _____ is shifting the epicenter there, where increased concern is focused on _____, due to its open and rapidly expanding _____ in the region that results in increasing _____ infection among young women and their babies.

4.   In the United States, by 1994, the Centers for Disease Control in Atlanta estimates _____ new cases of AIDS and well over _____ persons living with severe disease. The World Health Organization forcasts a minimum of _____ infected persons by the year 2000.

1. human hosts
2. HIV-2
3. sub-Saharan Central Africa
4. social-sexual changes
5. 12 million
6. pandemic
7. quarter of a million
8. sex industry
9. human immunodeficiency virus-1 (HIV-1)
10. Thailand
11. aggressive parasitic growth
12. 40 million
13. Uganda
14. half a million
15. simian immunodeficiency virus (SIV)
16. southeast Asia
17. virus
18. world travel

5.   Although the _____ of HIV infection varies, three distinct stages mark the relentless progression of the disease: (1) brief _____ with flu-like symptoms for about a week, followed by an extended _____ during asymptomatic incubation and constant viral growth.; (2) a beginning period of simple opportunistic illnesses called _____ and general signs of weakening immune function; and (3) _____ with accumulating illnesses such as tuberculosis, pneumonia, and Kaposi's sarcoma—a skin cancer. When the _____ finally kills enough _____ to overwhelm the weakened immune resistance to the disease complications, _____ follows.

6.   As in any major epidemic, the U.S. Public Health Service (PHS) has the major overall task of _____ the disease spread. Thus in the AIDS crisis, PHS is carrying out responsibilities in two major areas: (1) _____ including testing and counseling; and _____ through interrupting its spread, vaccine research, and treatment.

7.   _____ is increasingly essential since AIDS is now reaching into all communities in some form, cutting short the lives of children, adolescents, and young adults in accelerating numbers. The Harvard Global AIDS Policy Coalition now estimates that by the year 2000 as many as _____ adults and more than _____ infants and children will be infected worldwide.

1. virus
2. final stage of AIDS
3. monitoring and stopping
4. "well" period of 8-10 years
5. community education and prevention
6. 10 million
7. individual clinical course
8. surveillance
9. 110 million
10. white cells (T cells)
11. community involvement
12. primary HIV infection
13. death
14. AIDS-related complex (ARC)

8.   HIV-1 and HIV-2 belong to a class of viruses called _____, due to their reverse transcription of RNA into DNA in the cell nucleus, which is then integrated into the _____. The virus has a protective outer covering and an inner shell containing small _____ of genetic material including nine genes, along with several _____ including the reverse transcriptase.

9.   After entering the body, the virus attaches to the host's actively replicating _____, major lymphocytes of the body's _____. There it integrates itself

219

into the host cell's _____, infecting and eventually killing the _____. Rapidly increasing masses of _____ erupt from the dying cells in _____ that immediately infect new cells.

1. RNA strands
2. immune system
3. small buds
4. host cells
5. retrovirus

6. DNA copying system
7. T-helper white blood cells
8. virus particles
9. host cell DNA
10. enzymes

10. Throughout the world, _____ is central to the epidemic spread of HIV and AIDS. An estimated _____ of HIV infection worldwide if due to heterosexual behavior, _____ to homosexual behavior, and a relatively smaller proportion to _____ with _____.

11. A growing concern is the increasing number of cases among _____ and the vertical _____ from _____ to their infants during the intrapartum period of _____ at birth. Worldwide studies of HIV-seropositive newborns indicate a _____ rate in about _____ of the newborns. These infected babies require _____ during the first year of life.

12. The group of persons at greatest risk of HIV infection are those sexually active _____ who do not consistently practice _____ sexual behavior. This behavior consists of (1) consistent and correct _____, and (2) avoidance of _____ and _____ for HIV infection.

13. Persons who practice _____ are at risk if they share _____. However, the risk of receiving a contaminated _____ for medical purposes is now eliminated since donors are screened and the public _____ has been thoroughly cleared of HIV infection by a rigorous _____.

1. adolescents and adults
2. blood transfusion
3. 30%
4. frequent hospitalization
5. sexual behavior
6. multiple partners

7. HIV-infected mothers
8. contaminated needles
9. condom protection
10. persons at risk
11. 71%
12. double-testing program

13. heterosexual women
14. donated blood supply
15. intravenous drug use
16. labor and delivery
17. 15%
18. responsible and safe
19. maternal-fetal transmission

Discussion Questions

1. What testing procedures are used in diagnosing HIV infection? Why are such rigorous testing procedures, including pre- and post-test counseling, so important?

2.   Describe the basic roles of nutrition in the HIV disease through its progressive stages. Give examples in each instance.

3.   What are the current basic goals of medical management of HIV infection in all its stages?

4.   Describe the initial evaluation of an HIV-infected patient? Why is care by a special AIDS team of professional health care specialists critical in beginning and continuing individual personal care? Describe the roles of each team member. Why must the patient always be a central team member?

5.   Lacking as yet a vaccine or cure, what antiretroviral drugs does medical management have available to use and how do they act on the life process of the virus? What side effects occur? What drug has been effectively used to stimulate appetite and help control body wasting?

Self-Test Questions

<u>True-False</u>
      Circle the "T" if a statement is true and write a brief rational for its accuracy. If it is false, circle the "F" and write the correct statement.

T F   1.   All patients diagnosed as HIV infected should be considered to be at nutritional risk.

T F   2.   Malnutrition and weight loss occur in varying degrees throughout the HIV-infection disease process.

T F   3.   The antianorexic drug *megesterol acetate* (Megase), used successfully in cancer therapy, has proved to have little effect in counteracting the severe anorexia and hence improving food intake and weight gain in many AIDS patients.

T F   4.   Drug-diet interactions and progressive effects of HIV infection contribute to malabsorption of nutrients and body wasting.

T F   5.   The general metabolic changes occurring in progressive AIDS stages do not contribute significantly to the ongoing body wasting.

T F   6.   All HIV-infected patients, at first contact with a health professional, should be referred to the AIDS team clinical dietitian for screening to evaluate the degree of any nutrition problems.

T F   7.   The AIDS patient's wishes and needs are ultimately paramount in various treatments and decisions about care.

Self-Test Questions

<u>Multiple Choice</u>

    Circle the letter in front of the correct answer. Then check your responses by the test key (Appendix, p 285). Now compare all the possible answers for each item and write the following brief statements: (1) rationale for the correct answer and (2) why each of the other responses are wrong.

1.   The overall basic goal of nutrition counseling with the AIDS patient is to:
   - a.   change food habits to include more key vitamins and minerals
   - b.   suggest ways of increasing protein food sources
   - c.   make the fewest possible changes in lifestyle and food patterns
   - d.   increase the energy intake

2.   Information and actions discussed in AIDS nutrition counseling should:
   - a.   be agreed upon with the patient
   - b.   proceed in manageable steps, as small as need be
   - c.   follow in order of complexity and difficulty
   - d.   help provide psychosocial support
   - e.   all of the above

3.   The structure and nature of all viruses makes them
   - a.   the ultimate parasites
   - b.   able to grow and multiply on their own
   - c.   vulnerable to common antiviral drugs
   - d.   widespread in any environment

4.   The clinical course of HIV infection:
   - (1)   is relatively short
   - (2)   varies substantially on an individual basis
   - (3)   follows the same basic stages in all patients
   - (4)   lasts about 15-20 years
   - a.   1 and 2
   - b.   3 and 4
   - c.   2 and 3
   - d.   2 and 4

5.   During the relatively long "well" period of HIV infection the virus is
   - a.   incubating and multiplying in special tissues
   - b.   weakening in strength
   - c.   infecting fewer white cells
   - d.   inactive

6.   Common symptoms observed during the pre-AIDS period called AIDS-related complex (ARC) include:
   - a.   persistent fatigue, thrush or other oral soreness, night sweats, remarkable headache

b. diarrhea, elevated temperature, unintentional weight loss, new skin rash

c. new or unusual cough, shortness of breath, unusual bruises or skin discoloration

d. all of the above

7. In the course of the HIV infection, the AIDS final stage of death occurs when the virus

a. Finally kills enough white T cells to overwhelm the weakened immune system resistance

b. Develops into a more powerful genetic strain

c. Creates a large amount of overwhelming toxins due to its multipled numbers

d. Mutates into a more deadly form with increased amounts of cell-destroying enzymes such as transcriptase

Learning Activities

Individual Project: Roles of Clinical Dietitian and Nurse on AIDS Care Team

Interview a clinical dietitian and nurse involved in care of AIDS patients concerning their roles in team care and any specific activities involved with individual clients. If possible, arrange to accompany them on a home visit or observe a clinic visit.

Individual or Small Group Project: Unproved Therapies for AIDS

Investigate and evaluate any alternative unproved therapies for AIDS to which persons with AIDS or their families may be particularly vulnerable. See the *To Probe Further* article, "Are AIDS Patients Targets of Nutritional Hucksters?" for reference.

Visit a health food store or pharmacy to find any products, supplements, or print materials that may make any claims for use by persons with AIDS. Research these claims and evaluate the product(s) or statements in light of your nutrition knowledge gained in your text readings and class discussion. Report your findings to the class.

Group Project: Nutritional Resources for AIDS

Collect available patient guides or resources from any AIDS clinics or programs in your community. Check with your city or county Public Health Department or special AIDS care center available. Write or call the National AIDS Information Clearing House, Post Office Box 6003, Rockville, Maryland 20850, telephone 1-800-458-5231. Communicate with an individual community AIDS resource center, such as ARIS Project, AIDS Support Services in Santa Clara County, 595 Millich Drive, Suite 104, Campbell, California 95008, or other such facility in your own community. Report your findings to the class.

Current Nutrition Issues

Read carefully the *Issues and Answers* article, "Special Consideration for Pediatric Patients with AIDS" (*Essentials of Nutrition and Diet Therapy*, ed 6, p 484); *Nutrition and Diet Therapy*, ed 7, p 717). Consider these inquiry questions:

1. How does chilldhood growth and development contribute to the impact of HIV infection in an infant or young child? Why are continuing nutrition assessments essential?

2. Why are increased protein and kcalories usually needed? Suggest ways you may supplement a child's diet to accomplish these increases.

3. Why would vitamins and minerals also need to to be increased?

4. Why would close attention be needed to any drugs being used?

5. Describe ways of handling or feeding formula, milk, foods and dishes to avoid contamination.

Chapter 25
NUTRITION AND CANCER

Chapter Focus

Nutrition is related to cancer in both prevention and therapy. In the area of prevention, nutrition relates to the environment and to the body's defense system. In the area of therapy, nutrition relates to medical treatment and rehabilitation. Hence, vigorous nutritional support is essential to both immune system integrity and the healing process.

Summary-Review Quiz

Fill in the blanks below with the appropriate number and word(s) from the list following each section. Each numbered word or phrase is used; some may be used more than once. When you have completed all the sections, check your answers for each blank by the test key (Appendix, p 285). Correct any mistakes and then review the entire chapter summary.

1.   The term _____ refers to a malignant tumor or _____ --new growth. Since there are many _____ and multiple _____, we would be more correct to use the term _____ for this great variety of _____.
2.   Tumor development is a _____ based in the _____ structure and function of _____, guided by the _____ in the controlling _____ material _____. But in this case normal _____ and reproduction has lost its _____ and the _____ has "gone wild."

1. causes	6. neoplasm	11. cell nucleus
2. cells	7. genetic code	12. neoplasms
3. gene control	8. growth process	13. normal
4. cancers	9. DNA	14. different forms
5. cell growth	10. cancer	

3.   Types of cancer tumors are classified by (1) _____ of originating tissue and (2) _____ of development according to _____ and invasion of tissue. Cancer development is related to the _____ in cells, tissues, and organ systems.
4.   A number of factors contribute to loss of _____ over normal _____ and hence to cancer cell development. These factors include (1) _____ of genes, which may then be _____ and brought out by some _____ agent; (2) _____, which interfere with structure or function of _____ genes; (3) _____ which damages chromosomes; and (4) tumor-inducing _____ which change _____ genes by acting as _____.

1. rate of growth
2. environmental
3. cell reproduction
4. radiation
5. inherited
6. aging process
7. regulatory
8. chemical carcinogens
9. primary site
10. parasites
11. mutation
12. viruses
13. stage
14. gene control

5.   Studies of cancer incidence show that it is _____ in our population, with U.S. rates being _____ than those of many other countries. Numerous epidemiologic factors such as _____, _____, and age have been associated with cancer development. For example, _____ cancer has been closely related to consumption of _____ here and worldwide.

6.   Loss of a central relation and other _____ also relate to cancer development, probably caused by _____ effects of such psychic trauma; (1) damage to the _____ and (2) _____ responses to anxiety states.

1. diet
2. stress factors
3. immune system
4. greater
5. breast
6. physiologic
7. hormonal
8. endemic
9. dietary fats
10. region

7.   Two major groups of special protective white blood cells, the _____, provide our _____ main defense against malignant cells; (1) _____ from the thymus gland, which activate _____ and _____ response and (2) _____, which produce special protein _____. Both types of defending cells derive from precursor cells in the _____.

8.   Nutritional support relates directly to (1) integrity of the _____ for combating malignancy and (2) protein synthesis and supply of the key _____ essential to the tissue _____.

1. phagocytes
2. bone marrow
3. immune system
4. healing process
5. inflammatory
6. T cells
7. antibodies
8. vitamins and minerals
9. lymphocytes
10. B cells

9.   Medical treatment for cancer takes three major forms: (1) _____ for early accessible tumors, (2) _____ for responsive safely targeted tumors, and (3) _____ with recently developed _____ agents.

10.   All of these treatment modes depend on vigorous _____ to (1) promote the general _____, (2) meet _____ demands of the disease process, (3) modify special _____ or _____ factors, and (4) develop _____ modes to assure optimal intake.

1. chemotherapy
2. nutritional support
3. nutrient
4. feeding
5. radiation
6. healing process
7. texture
8. surgery
9. hypermetabolic
10. antineoplastic

11.   Nutritional _____ must be designed to meet problems related to (1) the _____ process itself and (2) the _____ of the disease. Thus a strong nutritional _____ must fulfill two major goals in (1) meeting _____ demands and preventing _____ and (2) controlling disease _____ and treatment _____ by adapting _____ and feeding process according to _____ needs.

12.   Major nutritional problems during chemotherapy include (1) _____ caused by drug effect on mucosal cells, (2) _____ from bone marrow effects, and (3) general _____ effect on _____ and food tolerances.

1. hypermetabolic
2. individual
3. side effects
4. cancer
5. appetite
6. anemia
7. catabolism
8. medical treatment
9. systemic toxicity
10. symptoms
11. gastrointestinal symptoms
12. therapy
13. food forms
14. care plan

13.   Successful nutritional therapy is based on (1) comprehensive personal _____ to develop a realistic care plan and (2) optimal _____ intake to maintain positive _____.

14.   The nutritional treatment plan must meet increased needs for (1) sufficient _____ to supply energy demands and spare _____ for healing, (2) optimum _____ ratio to maintain positive _____ and prevent _____, (3) key _____ for increased metabolic regulation, and (4) sufficient _____ to replace _____ and dispose of metabolic products and _____.

1. protein
2. fluid
3. nutritional status
4. nitrogen balance
5. toxic drugs
6. nutrient and energy
7. catabolism
8. losses
9. nutritional assessment
10. protein/kcalories
11. vitamins and minerals
12. kcalories

15.   The method of _____ depends on the condition of the _____. If the gut works, _____ methods are used. Oral diet with _____ is desirable when possible. Adequate food intake may be hindered by general _____ or extreme _____, resulting in gross _____.

16.   Eating difficulties may come from problems in the _____ or _____ area. To meet individual needs and tolerances, food may be modified in _____, _____, or _____. If the gut works but the patient is unable to eat, enteral _____ may be used sometimes supplemented by

227

_____. If the gastrointestinal tract cannot be used and _____ is crucial, a form of _____ can be used. To meet short-term needs, _____ may be used alone. For greater long-term nutritional needs, _____ with _____ may be required.

1. enteral	10. mouth
2. malnutrition	11. concentrated nutrient solutions
3. temperature	12. feeding
4. parenteral feeding	13. total parenteral nutrition (TPN)
5. appetite loss	14. taste
6. peripheral parenteral nutrition (PPN)	15. nutritional support
7. gastrointestinal	16. cancer cachexia
8. individual patient	17. tube feeding
9. texture	18. nutrient supplementation

Discussion Questions

1. Why can a cancer patient not depend on the usual appetite and hunger mechanisms to regulate food intake? What suggestions can you give for improving food intake?

2. Why are highly toxic drugs used to treat cancer? What is the "cell or log kill" hypothesis governing use of these agents?

3. How may radiation therapy contribute to general malnutrition? How may nutritional therapy be managed to overcome such dangers?

4. What is cancer cachexia? Why is this a dangerous condition? What can be done about it?

Self-Test Questions

<u>True-False</u>
Circle the "T" if a statement is true and write a brief rationale for its accuracy. If it is false, circle the "F" and write the correct statement.

T F   1.   A cancer cell is unrelated to a normal cell.

T F   2.   Ribonucleic acid (RNA) is the genetic control agent in the cell nucleus.

T F   3.   Genes are specific sites along the chromosomes in the cell nucleus.

T F   4.   Chemical carcinogens are substances that change the structure or function of genes.

T F   5.   Cancer tumors arising from connective tissue are called carcinomas.

T F   6.   The incidence of cancer is not related to age.

T F   7.   Cancer-causing mutant genes may be inherited but their expression usually requires some added environmental agent.

T F   8.   Antigens are specialized protein components of our immune systems that protect us against disease.

T F   9.   Cancer surgery in the oropharyngeal area seldom requires diet modification in texture.

T F 10.   A cancer patient treated with a monoamineoxidase inhibitor drug requires a special low tyramine diet.

Multiple Choice

    Circle the letter in front of the correct answer. Then check your answers by the test key (Appendix, p 286). Now compare all the possible answers for each item and write the following brief statements: (1) rationale for the correct answer and (2) why each one of the other responses is incorrect.

1.   Special blood cells that are major components of the body's immune system are the:
    a.   erythrocytes
    b.   lymphocytes
    c.   platelets
    d.   antibodies

2.   Antineoplastic drugs used in chemotherapy include:
    a.   prochlorterazine (Compazine)
    b.   monoamineoxidase inhibitors
    c.   cyclophosphamide (Cytoxan)
    d.   hydrazine sulfate

3.   The underlying problem in cancer cachexia is an abnormality in metabolism of:
    a.   amino acids
    b.   fructose
    c.   fat
    d.   glucose

4.   Surgical treatment of pancreatic cancer may cause added problems requiring nutritional therapy. These problems include:
    a.   IDDM
    b.   hypertension
    c.   weight gain
    d.   loss of cell enzymes

5.   A serious primary problem resulting form prolonged vomiting from cancer chemotherapy relates to:
     a.   nitrogen balance
     b.   calcium balance
     c.   fluid and electrolyte balance
     d.   glucose balance
6.   Side effects of cancer chemotherapy that reflect the toxic effect of the drugs on rapidly reproducing cells include:
     a.   severe headaches
     b.   gastrointestinal symptoms
     c.   increased urination
     d.   decreased appetite
7.   Adequate high quality protein is essential in a cancer patient's diet to:
     a.   prevent catabolism
     b.   meet increased energy demands
     c.   prevent anabolism
     d.   stimulate hypermetabolism
8.   The nausea caused by cancer chemotherapy may be treated by small amounts of the following types of foods
     a.   liquid, hot foods
     b.   dry, spicy foods
     c.   warm, spicy foods
     d.   soft, cold foods

Learning Activities

Individual Project: Analysis of a Cancer Patient's Diet

Interview a cancer patient being treated by chemotherapy. Collect and analyze the following data:
     1.   specific drugs used, their specific main action and side effects
     2.   symptoms experienced by the patient
     3.   total food intake for 1 day
     4.   efforts made by patient to deal with any eating difficulties such as mouth problems, gastrointestinal problems, or loss of appetite
     5.   any supplements used

Calculate the protein and kilocalories in the day's food intake. Evaluate the protein/kcalorie ratio.

On the basis of your findings, outline a personal food plan for this patient. If possible, discuss the plan with the patient.

Individual or Group Project: Formula Survey

Visit a community or hospital pharmacy and survey the variety of liquid commercial food supplement products for oral use. Compare their nutrient values and costs.

Interview a hospital clinical dietitian and pharmacist to learn which commercial nutrient formulas are used as oral supplements to diets for cancer patients or as tube feedings. On what basis are these formulas selected? How are they prepared or served? If possible, visit a patient on such a formula to learn how well the formula is tolerated.

With the aid of the clinical dietitian and pharmacist, prepare a taste-testing session with other students and staff members. Compare palatability, nutrient values, and costs of a variety of formulas. Compare formulas designed for tube feeding. How do they differ?

Current Nutrition Issues

Read carefully the *Issues and Answers* article, "Toward the Prevention of Cancer" (*Essentials of Nutrition and Diet Therapy*, ed 6, p 501; *Nutrition and Diet Therapy*, ed 7, p 737). Consider these inquiry questions:

1. Why do you think persons continue to smoke or use other types of tobacco products when comprehensive research has clearly established the nicotine in tobacco as an addictive cancer-causing agent?

2. How does alcohol use relate to cancer as a risk factor?

3. What is the general attitude toward cancer in comparison with other chronic illness such as heart disease?

4. What cancer relationships with foods or food factors have been indicated or are under study? How do the NRC dietary guidelines for cancer prevention compare with the USDA Dietary Guidelines? (See Chapter 1 in your text.)

5. How would you evaluate each of these dietary guidelines for reducing the risk of cancer? How do they compare with your own food habits?

Chapter 26
NUTRITIONAL SUPPORT IN DISABLING
DISEASE AND REHABILITATION

Chapter Focus

Persons with severe disabling illness or injury carry physical, mental, and social burdens and require long-term specialized team care. Personal nutritional support is essential for the healing and restoring process. Positive nutritional care builds personal strengths and resources, based on individual needs and specific disease. Skilled and sensitive care combats malnutrition and retards the devastating disease consequences. Three major types of such health problems include *musculoskeletal disease*, *neuromuscular disease*, and *progressive neurologic disorders*.

Summary-Review Quiz

Fill in the blanks below with the appropriate number and word(s) from the list following each section. Each numbered word or phrase is used; some may be used more than once. When you have completed all the sections, check your answers for each blank by the test key (Appendix, p 287). Correct any mistakes and then review the entire chapter summary.

1. Positive supportive care for disabling conditions requires special _____. Two goals are basic in planning care: (1) to prevent further _____, and (2) to restore _____.

2. The complex process of care demands a strong _____, combining the unique resources of a number of skilled _____ to identify specific personal needs and provide _____.

3. Some not so apparent disabling conditions such as _____, _____, and _____ are _____ not easily observed by others. Persons with these less apparent conditions often lack the needed cues from others or _____ to assist their difficult personal process of _____.

1. person-centered care	7. health care specialists
2. team approach	8. diabetes
3. heart disease	9. team care
4. adaptation and healing	10. psychosocial support
5. invisible disabilities	11. kidney failure
6. potential function	12. disability

4. Special needs of disabled persons center on _____ and _____. The process of care for disabling injury or severe illness is _____, requiring adequate _____ resources and assistance if personal resources or _____

are limited. Everyday living problems may include need for an _____ or special equipment to maintain an _____ situation if at all possible.

5.   Other psychologic barriers from _____ problems require tremendous adjustment. These struggles may stem from loss of _____ as well as physical _____; rehabilitative processes may test both _____ and physical _____.   Each person's efforts must have sensitive _____ to meet _____.

1. self-esteem
2. independent living
3. inner strength
4. individual needs
5. long and costly
6. stamina
7. employment capabilities

8. practical and emotional
9. living situations
10. team support
11. attendant
12. economic problems
13. body trauma
14. financial

6.   Special needs of older disabled persons differ from those of younger persons, not only because the older population is _____, but also because of three life-changing effects of aging: (1) _____, (2)_____, and (3) _____.

7.   Adjustment to _____ is needed by many older persons, who may experience _____ from loss of _____ built on a lifetime of active involvement in a familiar working environment. They often need help in _____ to a changed life situation, as well as _____ to help find appropriate activities and _____ in which they can contribute their unique _____ to others.

1. personal adjustment
2. general physical decline
3. wisdom and skills
4. stressful disorientation
5. chronic illnesses

6. vocational programs
7. retirement
8. employment
9. self-identity
10. increasing

8.   In the 60 to 75 age group of "young-old" persons, most _____ needs relate to residual disabilities from chronic diseases of aging such as : (1) _____, (2) _____, (3) _____, or (4) _____.

9.   In addition, problems may be increased by damaging personal health behaviors such as: (1) _____, (2) _____, (3) _____, and (4) _____.   Early _____ efforts help prevent _____, avoid _____, and restore reasonable _____.

1. alcoholism
2. disability
3. function
4. stroke
5. excessive diet high in fat and salt
6. heart disease
7. complications
8. hypertension
9. smoking
10. cancer
11. rehabilitation
12. lack of physical activity

10. In the 75 to 85+ age group of "old-old" persons, physical decline and _____ increases markedly, largely due to _____, chronic _____, problems with _____ , increased _____ and interactions. Often there are several chronic conditions, numerous _____, and various medical treatments. Minor disabilities easily become _____. _____ care is essential in _____, depression, _____ decline, infections, and _____ from poor nutrition and fad diets.

1. nutrient-energy deficits
2. different medications
3. chronic diseases
4. sensory
5. drug reactions
6. locomotion and perception
7. nutritional
8. falls and fractures
9. major handicaps
10. disability
11. brain failure

11. In rehabilitation two basic goals of supporting nutritional care are _____ and _____. _____ involves hard work, and thus the diet must supply sufficient _____ to meet the total _____ and physical activity energy demands. To prevent obesity excessive _____ should be avoided.

12. Sufficient _____ is required to maintain strong tissue structure and function, especially to protect against the _____ that usually follows severe trauma such as _____. High _____ also helps prevent _____ during long periods of immobility in bed patients, infections, and negative _____.

13. To meet critical energy needs, optimal dietary _____ serves as the body's major source of essential fuel. Sufficient _____ foods also help spare _____ for its essential _____ function. Sufficient moderate amounts of _____ must supply _____, the essential fatty acid, as well as contribute a secondary fuel source. A diet containing about _____ of its total kcalories as _____ is sufficient. An optimal intake of _____ and _____ maintains increased metabolic activity and _____.

1. nitrogen balance
2. fat
3. quality protein
4. vitamins
5. tissue reserves
6. kcalories
7. linoleic acid
8. spinal cord injury
9. physical therapy
10. 30%
11. restoration of eating ability
12. decubitus ulcers
13. basal metabolic
14. minerals
15. carbohydrate
16. prevention of malnutrition
17. tissue building
18. energy intake
19. catabolism

14. Three examples of disabling conditions from musculoskeletal disease are: (1) rheumatoid _____, which occurs mainly in young adults; (2) _____, which affects middle and older adults, and (3)_____, which mainly affects _____ women.

15. Rheumatoid _____ is a severe type of _____ disease that attacks the _____ of joints, causing deformity and destruction. These changes limit ability to _____, shop for food, or _____.

16. A milder adult form of _____, correctly called _____, mainly affects joints of the _____ and may become disabling with aging. However, damaged joints can be surgically replaced by _____.

17. The common metabolic bone disorder _____ affects _____ and increasing disability from _____, especially in the elderly.

1. autoimmune	5. osteoarthritis	9. self-feed
2. bone fractures	6. hands, knees, and hips	10. osteoporosis
3. synosheaths	7. degenerative joint disease	11. arthroplasty
4. prepare food	8. bone calcium loss	12. post-menopausal
		13. arthritis

18. Traumatic injury of the _____ is the leading cause of death in the first four decades of life in the United States, and the _____ leading cause of death for all ages. With current advances in _____ more persons survive severe _____ injury, but sustain serious _____ requiring extended _____.

19. Early nutrition support centers on combatting the initial _____ phase and its increasing tissue protein _____ that depletes _____. The large amount of _____ required may be supplied by _____ or _____ means. Individual follow-up rehabilitation is provided according to _____ of abilities in _____ including _____ and eating.

1. rehabilitation	6. third	11. food preparation
2. catabolism	7. protein and kcalories	12. brain and spinal cord
3. daily living skills	8. emergency medicine	13. lean body mass
4. disability	9. parenteral	14. needs assessment
5. enteral	10. hypermetabolic	

20. Neuromuscular conditions occurring during childhood cause various developmental difficulties such as: (1) _____, a general term for nonprogressive disorders of _____, either _____ or _____ in nature; (2) _____, a disorder in which abnormal _____ activity in the brain causes _____; and (3) _____, a congenital defect in formation of the spine. In each type of disorder respectively, nutritional care focuses mainly on: (1) _____ due to oral motor disfunction; (2) meeting _____ and drug side-effects, or problems such as intractable disease in young children that resists usual _____ and is sometimes managed by a special _____; and (3) dealing with _____, and with

_____ due to limited _____ and to _____ by parents or other caregivers as compensating rewards.

1. athetoid
2. electrical
3. normal growth needs
4. muscle control
5. growth retardation

6. epilepsy
7. physical activity
8. feeding problems
9. spina bifida
10. spastic

11. drug therapy
12. overfeeding
13. recurrent transient seizures
14. obesity
15. cerebral palsy
16. ketogenic diet

Matching: Progressive Neurologic Disorders

Write the correct disease name and letter for its corresponding definition and care in each of the numbered blanks below. Compare your responses with the answer key (Appendix, p 288). Correct any errors and review the related discussion in your textbook.

_____ 1. A rare autoimmune reaction following a viral infection bringing on acute nerve inflammation in which the myelin sheath covering the nerve axons deteriorates, causing loss of nerve conduction and varying degrees of paralysis; enteral or parenteral nutrition support may be needed in early acute phases; respiratory distress may require ventilator assistance and use of increased fat to carbohydrate dietary ratio for needed energy fuel; soft textured foods in early oral feedings ease chewing-swallowing problems.

_____ 2. Degeneration of basal ganglia cells in the brain that produce the neurotransmitter dopamine which controls flow of nerve signals to muscles and thus regulates muscle function; drug therapy with levodopa supplies needed dopamine and slows disease progression; nutritional care centers on related drug effects such as nausea, eating problems due to hand tremor, and malnutrition.

_____ 3. Progressive disease of the central nervous system in which scattered patches of nerve-insulating myelin are destroyed and replaced by non-functioning scar tissue, interfering with normal transmission of nerve impulses; precise cause unknown, but its autoimmune nature causes body's defense system to treat myelin tissue as a foreign tissue and gradually sets out to destroy it; the new genetically engineered drug beta-interferon (Betaseron) helps regulate the immune system; diet is generally low in fat.

_____ 4. A progressive dementia in which nerve cells in the brain degenerate and the brain substance shrinks; specific cause unknown and diagnosis can only be verified after death; still no way of stopping the inevitable progression of years of mental and personal decline until death; major nutritional goal is to prevent malnutrition and devise ways of helping with feeding problems.

236

_____ 5. An uncommon genetic disease in which degeneration of basal ganglia cells of the brain results in rapid, jerky, involuntary movements and progressive mental impairment; gene recently is discovered but there is still no cure; nutritional care centers on providing sufficient energy and nutrient intake to prevent malnutrition and excess weight loss.

_____ 6. Relentless genetic nerve degeneration that progresses to affect muscles of breathing and swallowing, usually killing its victims in about 3 years; nutritional care focuses on increased energy and nutrient intake, eating assistance for frequent small meals, then enteral-parenteral support in advanced stages.

_____ 7. Rare progressive neuromuscular disease, an autoimmune disorder, in which the body's immune system gradually destroys the muscle receptors that pick up nerve impulses, thus causing the muscles to respond only weakly or not at all; the resulting paralysis effects bring problems in speaking, eating, and other activities of daily living, or in severe cases weakened chest muscles cause breathing difficulties; drug therapy increases amount of the neurotransmitter acetylcholine to nerve endings; nutritional care focuses on optimal nutrition in form most easily tolerated, with supplemental enteral support as needed.

a. Parkinson's disease
b. Huntington's chorea
c. Guillian-Barré syndrome
d. Amyotrophic lateral sclerosis
e. multiple sclerosis
f. myasthenia gravis
g. Alzheimer's disease

Discussion Questions

1. Relate protein intake to the three stages of catabolism following severe tissue trauma. What is the effect of negative nitrogen balance? How does optimal protein intake help prevent catabolic injury?

2. Why is a good supply of carbohydrate important for sound nutritional support in disabling conditions, both in relation to energy and to protein? What is the comparative role of fat?

3. Why are increased amounts of vitamins and minerals needed in hypermetabolic conditions?

4. Describe some self-help devices used in helping disabled persons restore independent eating ability. Why is this ability important, especially in childhood forms of rheumatoid arthritis.

Self-Test Questions

True-False
Circle the "T" if the statement is true and write a brief rationale for its accuracy. If it is false, circle the "F" and write the correct statement.

T F 1. The complex and complicated rehabilitation process following disabling injury or disease requires a strong team approach, including professional specialists, patient, and family.

T F 2. The number of disabled Americans is decreasing so the cost of their long-term care is covered by the Federal Rehabilitation Act.

T F 3. The health of older persons improves after retirement at age 65.

T F 4. The U.S. Rehabilitation Services estimates that after age 65, one in three Americans will be disabled.

T F 5. Catabolism always follows major body trauma such as spinal cord injury.

T F 6. Post-injury energy needs are usually decreased during rehabilitation.

T F 7. Fat should supply only about 15% of the diet's total kilocalories during rehabilitation to avoid obesity.

T F 8. The normal vitamin-mineral RDA standards for age and sex are adequate for most disabled persons.

T F 9. The rehabilitation goal for each disabled person is to achieve as much daily-living independence as possible.

T F 10. Childhood rheumatoid arthritis affects only the small joints of the upper extremities.

T F 11. Marked disability with osteoarthritis is common.

Multiple Choice
Circle the letter in front of the correct answer. Then check your answers by the test key (Appendix, p 288). Now compare all the possible answers for each item and write the following brief statemnts: (1) rationale for the correct answer and (2) why each one of the other responses is incorrect.

238

1. In the team approach to rehabilitative care of disabled persons the key member of the team is the:
   a. physician
   b. nutritionist
   c. physical therapist
   d. nurse
   e. patient

2. By the mid-1990s, the estimated numbers of disabled Americans will have:
   (1) increased
   (2) decreased
   (3) remained unchanged
   (4) include more elderly persons
   (5) include more young persons
   a. 2 and 4
   b. 3 and 5
   c. 1 and 4
   d. 3 and 4

3. Following illness, injury, or chronic disease, early rehabilitation efforts help to:
   a. prevent disability
   b. avoid complications
   c. restore reasonable function
   d. all of these

4. During the rehabilitation process, nutritional therapy for the disabled person includes which of the following dietary principles?
   (1) Low protein to avoid overtaxing the kidneys
   (2) High protein to prevent tissue catabolism
   (3) High carbohydrate to supply sufficient energy
   (4) Low carbohydrate to prevent obesity
   (5) High fat to supply needed kilocalories and prevent weight loss
   (6) Moderate fat to meet metabolic needs and energy demands
   a. 1, 3, and 5
   b. 2, 3, and 5
   c. 2, 3, and 6
   d. 1, 4, and 5

5. In planning a diet for a person with rheumatoid arthritis, which of the following factors need to be considered?
   a. Sufficient energy intake to meet increased metabolic needs and disease activity stress
   b. Variable protein intake based on individual nutritional status and disease activity
   c. Standard amounts of vitamins and minerals for age and sex
   d. All of these

6.   Conditions of muscular weakness or incoordination that involve feeding problems and require use of self-feeding devices or some degree of feeding assistance include:

        a. ALS
        b. CVA
        c. Parkinson's disease
        d. All of these

Learning Activities

Group Project: Community Rehabilitation Program

In partners or small groups, investigate any available community or regional rehabilitation center program. Contact the director or nutritionist, or other staff person, and make an appointment to learn about their program. Organize your field trip and interview ahead, using the following points as a guide for discussions:

1.   Nature of the overall program, its history, philosophy and goals for treatment, and their experience with extent of rehabilitation problems in the community, region, or state.

2.   Types of problems the center is treating and the nature of the individual treatment program, roles of the therapists, patient, and family.

3.   In particular, interview the nutritionist about the center's nutrition program, its objectives, goals, methods, activities, results, and means of evaluation. What are the nutrition education activities? Collect samples of the nutrition education materials used, if available. What problems or needs does the program have? How is the staff trying to meet these needs? Is there any way you or your class may make a contribution of time, goods, or services to help or learn more about the program.

4.   If possible, interview a rehabilitation patient, or a disabled person you may know, about personal experiences and problems they have encountered living with a disability. Include a basic diet history, a 24-hour recall of food intake (see Chapter 17), and assess its general nutritional value by calculating the energy and protein intake. If a computer and nutrition assessment program is available, do a full nutritional analysis and compare the results with the person's nutritional needs.

5.   If a Center for Independent Living is available in your community to aid disabled persons, include a study of its program in your investigation. Compare its structure, organization and programs, with that of the community or regional rehabilitation center. What purposes does each serve?

Plan an oral report of your findings to your class as a basis for general class discussion. Include a display of any materials you have gathered.

Current Nutrition Issues

Read carefully the *Issues and Answers* article "Independent Living vs The Kindness of Strangers" (Essentials of Nutrition and Diet Therapy, ed 6, p 521; Nutrition and Diet Therapy, ed 7, p 760). Consider these inquiry questions:

1. What is the current legislative and enforcement status of the Federal Rehabilitation Act? Are these regulations established at the state level? What is the status of the regulations in your state and community?

2. Why do you think the total number of disabled persons in America has been rising during the past decade? What are the projections for the future? What are some leading causes of disability in America? In your community?

3. What have you observed in your community about the attitudes and treatment of disabled persons in regard to opportunities for education, employment, access to public facilities? How do you think some of these problems may be solved?

4. What continued problems do you see in general public policy concerning physical or mental disability for the future? Can you suggest any helpful approach to these problems?

APPENDIX
TEST KEY: Answers to Summary-Review Quizzes
and
Self-Test Questions

Chapter 1: Nutrition and Health

Summary-Review Quiz

1. 12, 6, 1, 8, 4
2. 13, 10, 15, 7, 14, 2, 9, 11, 5, 3

3. 9, 2, 7, 3, 5
4. 1, 10, 6, 11, 8, 4

5. 6, 7, 9, 1, 5, 2, 7, 11
6. 3, 8, 10, 4

7. 11, 5, 8, 1, 12
8. 9, 2, 6, 7
9. 4, 3, 10

Self-Test Questions

<u>True-False</u>

1. **T** Social attitudes stem from pioneer traditions and a larger number of young persons in prior population; a move away from former extended family pattern to single nuclear family; current youth focus in services, goods, marketing, housing; ageism in jobs, mandatory retirement practices, fixed incomes. (See *Essentials*, Chapter 13)

2. **T** Habits of any kind have cultural and psychosocial roots. This is especially true of food habits because of their intimate personal meanings.

3. **F** Total population has increased but mobility and age-adjustment have changed, with the number of persons moving from place to place and size of older age group increasing rapidly. (See *Essentials*, Chapter 13)

4. **F** Metabolism of nutrients is always highly interrelated.

5. **F** Processing changes food form, affecting both nutrients and sensory characteristics, as well as safety.

6. **F** No single food as such contains all our needed nutrients; thus no food can be called a complete food. We need a variety of foods so that the fill food mix provides a complete diet.

Multiple-Choice

1. **b** The same basic nutrients are necessary for all human life; the amount varies in general population groups with age and body size as reflected in the RDA standards and in individuals according to reproduction cycle, state of health, or disease.
2. **b** Nutrients are various chemical elements and compounds, found in a wide variety of foods, whose metabolic functions vary specifically according to their chemical natures.
3. **a** A varied mixed diet, balanced in nutritive value, supplies the specific nutrients required by the body. In special conditions such as disease, age, debilitation, or physiologic stress, supplements to the diet may be needed.

Chapter 2: Carbohydrates

Summary-Review Quiz

1. 9, 5, 13, 11
2. 2, 7, 4, 8, 3, 12, 1, 10, 6

3. 13, 6, 17, 15, 1, 12, 18, 8, 2, 14, 3
4. 5, 16, 11, 7, 9, 4, 10

5. 12, 6, 3
6. 12, 1, 10, 9, 4
7. 2, 12, 7, 11, 5, 8

Self-Test Questions

True-False

1. **F** Only protein, of the three energy nutrients, contains nitrogen in addition to carbon, hydrogen, and oxygen.
2. **T** Starch in many food forms is a major staple carbohydrate fuel in diets throughout the world.
3. **T** Processed and refined foods have far less fiber than the primary food form, and dietary use of these processed foods has greatly increased.
4. **F** Lactose (milk sugar) has the least sweetness of the sugars.
5. **T** Blood sugar is glucose; sometimes called dextrose in solutions.
6. **F** Humans lack the digestive enzymes to break down dietary fiber, so it passes through the body as nondigestible residue.
7. **F** The small amounts of glycogen deposited in liver and muscle last only about 24 hours but are important because their constant daily turnover provides fuel back-up for energy during the brief fasting of sleep periods.

1.   **b**   Orange juice is a liquid form of simple sugar (fructose); it requires no mechanical or chemical digestion and can be immediately absorbed.

2.   **d**   Glucose is the refined fuel blood sugar. Starch and dextrins are polysaccharides and maltose is a disaccharide, all of which require further digestive breakdown before they are available as glucose.

3.   **c**   All the effective carbohydrate enzymes are located in the small intestine mucosa.

4.   **b**   The specific disaccharidase, lactase, breaks down the sugar lactose found in milk. Sucrase is the specific enzyme for sucrose, maltase for maltose, and amylase for starch.

5.   **c**   Carbohydrate digestion is achieved by intestinal disaccharidases and pancreatic amylase.

6.   **d**   Insulin controls glucose metabolism, although other hormones have interbalancing effects.

7.   **a**   Glucose is constantly being converted to liver and muscle glycogen as a rapidly turning over back-up energy source.

Chapter 3: Fats

Summary-Review Quiz

1.   6, 10, 7
2.   3, 8, 5
3.   1, 9, 12, 11, 2, 4

4.   12, 7, 5, 13, 14
5.   3, 10, 15, 3, 1, 11, 2, 6, 4, 9, 8

6.   7, 4, 9, 2, 11, 10, 3, 8
7.   6, 1, 5

8.   10, 15, 13, 6, 16, 1
9.   5, 16, 2, 10, 14, 2, 8, 4, 12
10.   12, 7, 9, 4, 11, 3

11.   10, 5, 12, 1, 11, 3
12.   4, 9, 6, 7, 3, 1
13.   4, 13, 8, 2, 14

Self-Test Questions

<u>True-False</u>
1. **T** Excess dietary cholesterol burdens the body's cholesterol breakdown and disposal and subsequent cholesterol balance, and in persons with lipid disorders contributes to elevated blood lipids.
2. **F** Corn oil is a polyunsaturated fat.
3. **F** Polyunsaturated fats come from plant sources.
4. **T** A diet using fats composed mainly of polyunsaturated fatty acids such as linoleic acid helps to lower elevated serum cholesterol levels.
5. **F** Bile cannot digest anything—it is not an enzyme. It is an emulsifier that prepares fats for digestion by the powerful lipase enzymes.
6. **F** End products of fat digestion are glycerol and fatty acids.
7. **T** Chylomicrons are lipoproteins formed in the intestinal wall after a meal to transport the exogenous dietary fat just consumed. The other lipoproteins are formed in the liver to transport endogenous fat to and from various body tissues.
8. **F** Fat has more than twice the energy (kcalorie) value of carbohydrate: fat fuel factor is 9, whereas that of carbohydrate is only 4.

<u>Multiple Choice</u>
1. **a** Triglyceride is the chemical name for fat whether it is in the body or in foods. Fatty acids, glycerol, and lipoproteins are products of fat digestion and metabolism in the body.
2. **c** Saturated fats, mainly from animal sources, are made up of component fatty acids having all their available bonds filled with hydrogen; so they are more dense—harder—than other fats. Polyunsaturated fats from plant sources have several double bonds unfilled with hydrogen, so are soft to liquid in physical form.
3. **b** Vegetable oil is an unsaturated fat, whereas the fat of dairy products is saturated animal fat.
4. **c** Bile, an essential emulsifier to prepare fat for digestion by pancreatic lipase and absorption, is produced in the liver and stored in the gallbladder.
5. **b** In fat digestion, each fatty acid removed is split off from the glycerol base with increasing difficulty so that about 75% of the total fat remains as di- and monoglycerides for absorption. Digestive enzymes break down nutrients and do not emulsify or synthesize (build) products.

Chapter 4: Proteins

Summary-Review Quiz

1. 12, 8, 4, 1, 14
2. 2, 11, 13, 6, 3, 10
3. 7, 9, 5

4. 12, 6, 15
5. 8, 4, 8, 10, 3, 2, 14, 7, 9, 1, 11, 5, 16, 13

6. 10, 5, 16, 2, 3, 13
7. 7, 15, 9, 1, 6, 14, 4, 12, 2, 11, 8

8. 14, 7, 5, 11, 16
9. 4, 15, 9
10. 1, 13, 6, 8, 2, 12, 10, 3

11. 9, 3, 12, 1, 10, 5
12. 4, 7, 11, 8, 2, 6, 8

13. 10, 4, 1, 12, 6, 9
14. 8, 4, 14, 3, 14, 2
15. 11, 5, 13, 7, 5

Self-Test Questions

<u>True-False</u>
1. **F** Complete proteins are found in animal foods—milk, egg, cheese, and meat.
2. **T** Tissue building is the primary protein function. Protein only participates as an energy fuel according to dietary supply of the primary fuels, carbohydrate and fat.
3. **F** Carbohydrates and fats, not proteins, are the body's main fuels.
4. **T** Proteins are essential to the tissue-healing process and proper function of the immune system.
5. **F** The American diet is relatively high in protein, about 25% of total kcalories or more.
6. **F** Infants and children require more protein per kilogram body weight to meet tissue growth needs.
7. **F** Total caloric need lessens in old age with reduced activity but adult protein needs remain about the same for tissue maintenance.
8. **T** Protein is the building material of all body structures.
9. **T** Protein-energy malnutrition is the primary world health problem.

10. **T** An ill person is often in negative nitrogen balance from the catabolic effects of disease.

11. **T** Rapid growth requires extra nitrogen storage in new tissue being built, a period of anabolism.

12. **T** In a debilitated state of negative nitrogen balance, a person lacks sufficient protein to synthesize immune system components such as antibodies or blood cell factors.

13. **T** Both cheese and meat are complete protein foods. Meat is only considered better than cheese because it is generally regarded as a high status or "strength-giving" food.

14. **F** All grains are incomplete proteins.

15. **T** Egg protein has an amino acid profile more nearly like that of human requirements than has meat.

Multiple Choice

1. **a** Here the term *essential* refers specifically to *dietary* essentiality because the body can only obtain these 9 amino acids from the diet.

2. **d** A food protein is called "complete" if it provides these 9 amino acids in sufficient amounts.

3. **b** Proteins are large complex molecules requiring an extensive system of active enzymes to break them down to their constituent amino acids. The initial gastric enzyme pepsin is activated by gastric hydrochloric acid.

4. **b** For absorption, amino acids require active transport using activated vitamin B_6 (B_6PO_4) as a carrier. Smaller molecules can move across membranes by osmosis (water molecules) or diffusion (solutes in water solution).

5. **d** Protein balance is a state of dynamic equilibrium (homeostasis) between anabolism (tissue build-up) and catabolism (tissue breakdown).

Chapter 5: Digestion, Absorption, and Metabolism

Summary-Review Quiz

1. 10, 3, 7, 1, 8, 6, 11, 10
2. 2, 5, 4, 12, 9

3. 10, 12, 8
4. 3, 5, 10, 6, 11, 1, 4, 9, 7, 2

5. 9, 4, 7, 1, 6, 12
6. 2, 11, 3, 8, 5
7. 10

8.   10, 1 12
9.   2, 11, 7, 5, 9
10.   3, 8, 6, 4

11.   9, 4, 7, 5, 12, 2
12.   7, 1, 10, 8, 6, 11, 8, 6, 3, 7

13.   11, 9, 5, 1, 12, 2, 10
14.   8, 14, 3
15.   7, 4, 13, 6, 4

16.   7, 4, 10, 6, 3
17.   1, 9, 5, 8, 2

Self-Test Questions

True-False

1.   **F**   The pyloric valve releases acid gastric contents into the duodenum. The ileocecal valve controls intestinal flow from the ileum (last section of the small intestine) into the cecum (first section of the large intestine).
2.   **F**   Tremendous absorbing surface area of small intestine provided by specialized structures: mucosal folds, villi, and microvilli.
3.   **T**   Many digestive enzymes are secreted in an inactive form and require an activating agent; e.g., major gastric protein-splitting enzyme is secreted as inactive pepsinogen and requires gastric hydrochloric acid for change to active pepsin.
4.   **F**   Bile is an emulsifier, not an enzyme. It prepares fat for digestion by lipase enzymes.
5.   **F**   Enzyme action is always specific for its specific substrate. It won't "fit" anything else.
6.   **T**   The "gastrointestinal circulation" interfaces with the blood circulation and makes overall digestion, absorption, and metabolism possible.
7.   **F**   Bile (from gallbladder) and pancreatic enzymes enter the small intestine at the biliary duct.
8.   **T**   Presence of fat in the duodenum triggers release of the local hormone cholecystokinin, which in turn stimulates gallbladder to release needed bile.

Multiple Choice

1.   **d**   Peristalsis is the overall synchronized muscle action moving food mass alone the gastrointestinal tract by numerous coordinated individual nerve-muscle actions.

2.   c   Hormones, nreve network, and sensory stimuli (sight, smell, taste of food) trigger gastrointestinal secretions in an integrated manner, then the enzymes secreted digest the food nutrients.

3.   c   Mucus is only an important lubricating agent; it has no chemical properties to activate, acidify, or emulsify.

4.   b   The pyloric valve is located between the stomach and the small intestine. Sphincter muscles at other strategic points also act as valves to control food mass passage: gastroesophageal, ileocecal, and anal.

5.   b   Pepsin is secreted in inactive form by the chief cells in the gastric mucosa and activated by gastric hydrochloric acid present to begin the digestion of proteins.

6.   d   Fat in a food mix retards stomach-emptying time.

7.   d   Bile is secreted in watery form by the liver, condensed and stored by the gallbladder, and released as needed to emulsify fats for digestion by lipase.

8.   b   This constant bile-conserving circulation between the liver, gallbladder, and gastrointestinal tract serves the needs of all organs involved. Its efficiency is evident—of the 20 to 30 g of needed bile acids circulated daily to aid digestion and absorption of fats, only about 0.8 g is lost in the feces and requires replacement; the large portion is constantly reabsorbed to maintain the regular circulation.

9.   a   Because they are insoluble in water, fats go first into the lymphatic system (villi lacteals) and finally into portal circulation via the thoracic duct.

10. d   The final lipase in the series, lipoprotein lipase, acts on the absorbed post-meal, high-fat chylomicrons to clear them rapidly from the blood.

Chapter 6: Energy Balance and Weight Management

Summary-Review Quiz

Energy Balance
1.   12, 7, 11, 4, 8, 8, 5, 10, 6
2.   1, 2, 9, 2, 3, 10

3.   11, 4, 9, 1, 3, 6, 10, 13, 7, 2, 14, 5, 12, 8

4.   9, 5, 11, 1, 7, 13, 3
5.   2, 14, 4, 8, 6, 12, 10

6.   15, 5, 9
7.   1, 6, 18, 1, 2, 6
8.   3, 13, 8, 17, 4, 10, 14, 11, 7, 12, 16

9.   4, 2, 11, 1, 9, 6, 10
10.   3, 12, 7, 5, 8

<u>Weight Management</u>
1.   11, 7, 1, 4, 13, 8, 3, 12, 9
2.   5, 6, 2, 10

3.   13, 4, 10, 7, 1, 12, 3, 8, 14, 5, 2, 9, 6, 11

4.   2, 6, 14, 3, 8
5.   1, 11, 4, 12, 11, 13, 5, 10, 9, 7

6.   11, 7, 3
7.   1, 12, 5, 8, 4, 9, 6, 2, 10

8.   9, 5, 1, 12, 3, 10, 7, 6, 11, 2, 8, 4

9.   10, 6, 14, 1, 12, 7, 3, 1, 8
10.   5, 11, 2, 13, 4, 9, 5

Self-Test Questions

<u>True-False</u>
1.   **F**   Lowered food intake and its metabolic workload reduces the body's basal metabolic rate.
2.   **T**   Both pregnancy and lactation raise the BMR but lactation also entails the energy value of milk itself constantly being removed and replaced.
3.   **F**   Disease stimulates counteracting body defense mechanisms as well as influences ongoing tissue metabolism, often producing a hypermetabolic state.
4.   **F**   Glycogen provides a short-term energy reserve lasting about 24 hours.
5.   **F**   Catabolism is the process of breaking down tissue and metabolic products. The process of anabolism builds new tissue and metabolic products.
6.   **F**   Enzyme action is always specific for a specific substrate.
7.   **F**   Phosphate bonds such as ATP are high-energy bonds. Hydrogen bonds are weaker, easily broken bonds.
8.   **T**   Electrical energy of brain and nervous activity is measured in tests such as the electroencephlogram (EEG).
9.   **T**   After food energy is transferred to high-energy bonds in metabolic products such as ATP, the remaining water from metabolism is excreted by the kidneys, skin, as vapor by the lungs, and in fecal elimination. The remaining carbon dioxide is exhaled by the lungs.
10.   **F**   Kilocalorie is simply a unit of measuring potential energy in the food we eat.

11. F Appetite is a learned response influenced by many factors in one's life.
12. T Satiety is feeling of fullness or sense of having had enough to eat.
13. F Hunger is a basic biologic drive.
14. F Genetics provides a predisposition for a larger number of fat cells in developmental years, but excess eating habits add to the amount of fat deposits.
15. T Exercise not only expends energy but also helps establish a lower set-point for adipose tissue formation.
16. F A girl has higher fat deposits, especially in the abdominal pelvic girdle, as preparation for potential reproductive needs.
17. T Lower kilocalorie values are likely to be inadequate in meeting nutrient needs.
18. F Foods are exchanged only within their own group of equivalent foods.
19. F Often for some persons multiple small meals are more effective than three larger ones with no snacks.

Multiple Choice
1. a The kilocalorie is a measure of heat energy resulting from the "burning" of our food by our bodies.
2. b The small but rapidly growing young infant requires more energy per kilogram body weight to meet rapid growth demands.
3. c Hyperthyroidism stimulates BMR, demanding more energy supply.
4. d Fat has the highest fuel factor: 9 kcal/g.
5. c 2 g protein x 4 kcal = 8 kcal; 15 g carbohydrate x 4 kcal = 60 kcal; total 68 kcal.

Chapter 7: Vitamins

Summary-Review Quiz

Fat-Soluble Vitamins
1. 10, 4, 13, 6, 3, 14
2. 1, 11, 7
3. 12, 2, 8, 5, 9

4. 11, 3, 13, 1, 6, 14, 11, 5, 10, 9, 8, 2, 7
5. 4, 8, 12

6. 9, 4, 2, 11
7. 12, 3, 5, 1, 8, 7, 10, 6

8.   10, 12, 19, 1, 7, 6, 1, 14, 4, 8
9.   16, 9, 2, 4, 20, 11
10.   13, 5, 12, 18, 3, 17

11.   11, 4, 7, 2, 5, 10, 1, 9, 3, 8, 6

12.   9, 2, 12, 4, 6, 1
13.   12, 14, 3, 13, 8, 2, 4, 11, 7, 5, 10

Self-Test Questions

<u>True-False</u>
1.   **F**   Coenzymes, like their enzyme partners, are specific agents for control of specific metabolic reactions.
2.   **F**   Carotene, a plant pigment, is a precursor of vitamin A and is converted to the vitamin in the body.
3.   **F**   Vitamin A is fat-soluble, hence found in the fat part of milk.
4.   **F**   Visual purple (rhodopsin) is associated with light-dark adaptations of the eye.
5.   **T**   Vitamin D hormone facilitates absorption of calcium and phosphorus and their use in bone-building.
6.   **T**   A cholesterol compound in the skin is irradiated to form the vitamin D precursor that is subsequently metabolized to an intermediate form in the liver and then finally activated by special enzymes in the kidney to the physiologically active hormone.
7.   **F**   Vitamin A especially has potential toxicity because of its large storage capacity in the liver.
8.   **T**   These are the two types of substances from which vitamin K was originally isolated and formed.

<u>Multiple Choice</u>
1.   **b**   Carrots and green vegetables contain carotene; butterfat contains vitamin A. Nonfat milk naturally lacks the vitamin A-rich cream portion; oranges and tomatoes lack the vitamin precursor beta-carotene.
2.   **d**   Bile is needed for digestion and absorption of all fat and fat-soluble materials.
3.   **c**   The potential toxicity of vitamin A megadoses is enhanced by its extended liver storage capacity.
4.   **a**   Vitamin A is a key component of visual purple (rhodopsin), the retinal compound controlling the eye's vision adaptation to light and dark.
5.   **c**   Sunlight irradiation of a precursor cholesterol compound in the skin forms the initial stage of vitamin D, which is then changed in the liver to an intermediate form and finally activated by enzymes in the kidneys.

6.   **b**   The antioxidant properties of vitamin E enable it to protect lipid cell membrane structures from oxidation by free cell radicals.

7.   **d**   Vitamin K occurs in some food sources such as cheese, egg, liver, and green vegetables, but our main source is synthesis by intestinal bacteria.

Water-Soluble Vitamins
1.   8, 6, 5, 2, 10, 1, 4, 7
2.   8, 3, 9

3.   13, 5, 16, 2, 12, 7, 17, 1, 15, 3
4.   7, 9, 11, 4, 14
5.   6, 8, 10

6.   12, 6, 15, 1, 1, 4, 18, 8, 11, 16, 2
7.   5, 12, 3, 17, 14, 10, 7, 13, 9

8.   10, 5, 1, 12, 4, 7, 2, 12, 11, 6, 9, 8, 3

9.   6, 10, 3, 12, 1, 8, 12
10.   4, 10, 7, 11, 2, 5, 9

11.   9, 3, 14, 3, 6, 12, 5, 8, 1, 7, 11
12.   2, 10, 13, 4

13.   10, 3, 6, 12, 4, 7, 1, 2, 11, 8, 5, 9

14.   11, 5, 18, 2, 16, 8
15.   1, 15, 9, 12, 14, 12, 3, 14, 10, 4, 17, 9, 6, 1, 13, 7

Self-Test Questions

True-False
1.   **T**   Vitamin C helps build ground substance into connective tissue by deposits of intercellular cemenying material.
2.   **F**   Vitamin is not stored in any special oragn but a general overall tissue saturation level is maintained to meet body needs for tissue integrity.
3.   **F**   Vitamin C is unstable and easily oxidized.
4.   **T**   Thiamin is a necessary coenzyme factor in energy metabolism.
5.   **F**   Thiamin occurs naturally in few foods but is added to grain products that are enriched.
6.   **T**   Each quart of milk contains 2 mg of riboflavin as a milk pigment.
7.   **F**   The disease pellagra is associated with a deficiency of niacin.
8.   **F**   Pyridoxine (B_6) is a carrier for the absorption of amino acids.

9.	T	Pantothenic acid is a component of coenzyme A, which forms acetyl CoA, a central activating compound in cell metabolism.

10.	F	Vitamin B_{12} occurs only in animal food sources. Deficiences have been found only among strict vegans who use no B_{12} supplement.

Multiple Choice

1.	c	Vitamin C is a simple water-soluble compound (similar in structure to glucose) not stored in the body, so excess amounts above general tissue needs are excreted.

2.	d	The cementing effect of vitamin C develops ground substance into collagen-type connective tissues and membranes. Vitamin E protects the lipid matrix of cell membrances, vitamin K is essential for blood clotting, and vitamin D hormone facilitates calcium and phosphorus absorption and metabolism.

3.	d	Main source of vitamin C is citrus fruit with additional amounts available in a variety of vegetables and other fruits.

4.	b	Muscle function in general is diminished by a thiamin deficiency, because of depressed energy metabolism. Nerve irritation of alcoholism (delerium tremens) is related to insufficient lipid myelin sheath on nerve fibers caused by lack of thiamin coenzyme.

5.	c	Lack of thiamin coenzyme contributes to neurologic problems. Vitamin A deficiency is associated with vision problems, vitamin D hormone deficiency with bone disease, and vitamin C deficiency with hemorrhagic disorders.

6.	a	Intrinsic factor, a component of the gastric secretions activated by hydrochloric acid, is necessary for vitamin B_{12} absorption.

Chapter 8: Minerals

Summary-Review Quiz

Major Minerals
1.	13, 5, 16, 1
2.	18, 9, 3, 7, 20, 12, 4, 9, 17, 14, 2, 19, 4, 9, 10, 6, 15, 11, 8

3.	9, 4, 11, 6, 1, 8, 2, 12
4.	3, 11, 5, 10, 7

5.	9, 5, 12, 3, 10, 1
6.	6, 11, 6, 2, 7, 3, 8, 11, 4, 8

7.	7, 2, 4, 10, 1, 6, 5, 9, 8, 3

8.   14, 14, 7, 17, 1, 11, 5, 16, 2, 20, 4
9.   9, 13, 3, 15, 19, 8
10.   18, 12, 6, 10

11.   12, 9, 6, 6, 16, 2, 14, 8, 4
12.   16, 7, 18, 1, 11, 5
13.   17, 13, 15, 15, 10, 3

Trace Elements
1.   8, 3, 1, 10, 5, 2
2.   3, 9, 9, 7, 4, 9, 6, 9, 3

3.   11, 2, 8, 11, 5, 12, 4, 9, 1, 8, 6
4.   10, 7, 3

5.   12, 3, 16, 7, 1, 10, 6
6.   4, 14, 2, 5, 14, 8, 15, 11, 13, 9

7.   11, 6, 8, 2, 6, 12, 4, 8, 6, 1, 3, 9, 5, 10, 7

8.   10, 4, 8, 2, 12
9.   1, 7, 6, 3, 5, 11, 9

10.   9, 5, 12, 2, 6, 1, 8, 10, 3
11   4, 7, 11

Water-Electrolyte Balance
1.   9, 5, 12
2.   1, 14, 3, 7, 13
3.   2, 10, 4, 11, 8, 6

4.   11, 4, 13, 7, 9, 5, 14, 3, 8, 2
5.   12, 10, 6, 1

6.   12, 6, 15, 9, 3, 14, 12, 1, 18
7.   2, 10, 7, 16, 4, 13, 5, 11, 13, 17, 11, 8

8.   5, 10, 5, 1, 7, 10, 3
9.   6, 2, 4, 8, 9

10.   9, 4, 1, 3, 6, 2, 14, 12, 3
11.   8, 11, 13, 5, 10, 7

Self-Test Questions

<u>True-False</u>
1. **T**   Lower pH (increased acidity) favors solubility of calcium and thus its absorption, mainly in first section (duodenum) of the small intestine where the food mass is still acidic from the gastric hydrochloric acid.
2. **F**   Only about 10% to 30% of the calcium in the average diet is absorbed.
3. **T**   The bone and serum calcium compartments are constantly interchanging according to need and physiologic stress factors.
4. **T**   Generally we need only about 1.0 to 1.5 g sodium/day, but the average American diet usually far exceeds this amount from salt seasoning of food and the extensive use of salt and other sodium compounds in processed foods.
5. **F**   Edema is a state of excess tissue fluid.
6. **T**   As the major anion in extracellular fluid (ECF), Cl^- balances with Na^+, the major ECF cation.
7. **T**   The important structural sulfur bond is —SH.
8. **F**   Control of iron balance occurs at the point of absorption by the ferritin mechanism, where only about 10% to 30% of all the ingested iron is absorbed.
9. **T**   Liver is the main storage organ for a number of the body nutrients, including iron.
10. **F**   The trace element iron is not widespread in food sources, so iron-deficiency anemia is a prevalent health problem.
11. **T**   Vitamin C aids iron absorption by its reducing action and effect on acidity level required to prepare iron for absorption and body use.
12. **F**   The body avidly conserves and recycles its iron from hemoglobin of old red blood cells.
13. **F**   Nutritional anemia is caused by an iron deficiency.
14. **F**   Regular cow's milk has little or no iron content. Commercial infant formulas are iron enriched. Breast milk contains iron.
15. **F**   The only function of iodine is in thyroxine synthesis.
16. **F**   Thyroxine is synthesized by the thyroid gland.
17. **T**   Fluoride protects teeth from the acid erosion of bacterial action on food adhering to the teeth.

<u>Multiple Choice</u>
1. **d**   Vitamin D hormone and parathyroid hormone interact to control normal calcium balance at points of absorption, bone deposit and withdrawal, and renal excretion.
2. **c**   Phosphorus is a vital component of the activating and energy-binding compound adenosine triphosphate (ATP) in cell metabolism.
3. **a**   The necessary pH (acidity) for iron reduction to the necessary form for absorption is provided by gastric hydrochloric acid and vitamin C.

4.   **b**   The currently reduced incidence of dental caries is largely the result of the extended fluoridation of public water supplies.

Matching: Water-Electrolyte Balance
1.   k
2.   g
3.   n
4.   a
5.   l
6.   b
7.   f
8.   h
9.   i
10.   q
11.   d
12.   p
13.   j
14.   c
15.   e
16.   m
17.   o
18.   r

Chapter 9: The Food Environment and Food Habits

Summary-Review Quiz

Food Environment
1.   11, 6, 9, 1, 14
2.   4, 8, 13
3.   9, 2, 12, 5, 3, 10, 7

4.   11, 7, 14, 1, 9, 4, 13, 2
5.   12, 5, 8, 6, 10, 3

6.   8, 3, 12, 1, 10
7.   2, 11, 5, 7, 4, 9, 6

Food Habits
1.   12, 6, 15
2.   1, 8, 18, 4, 17, 13, 7
3.   16, 9, 3
4.   10, 10, 14, 5, 11, 2

5.   9, 3, 12, 6, 1, 10
6.   2, 7, 5, 4, 11, 8

7.   9, 12, 1, 5, 10, 7, 2, 11, 6
8.   3, 8, 4

9.   11, 2, 12, 6, 10, 4
10.   1, 7, 3, 9, 3, 9, 1, 8, 5

11.   8, 3, 17, 16, 12, 7, 18
12.   13, 9, 4, 1, 5, 14, 20, 11, 19
13.   10, 15, 6, 2

Self-Test Questions

True-False

1.   F   Pockets of hard-core poverty and malnutrition exist in urban centers and in depressed small town and rural areas, and additional families caught in newly depressed industries are also malnourished.
2.   F   Governing policies establish regulations controlling export and distribution of available food at national and local levels.
3.   F   In the highly competitive food market, new items are constantly being developed.
4.   T   The USDA and FDA have the responsibility by law to monitor and regulate the use of pesticides and food additives.
5.   F   Food habits are learned behaviors resulting from many influences in our lives.
6.   T   These four factors largely determine status in our society.
7.   T   Social lifestyles change constantly, slowly, or rapidly, depending on value changes in a society.
8.   T   Eating assumes many social relationships because of family and social influences throughout life.
9.   F   High status foods usually have little relation to their nutritional value but contribute more to esteem because of cost, availability, or desirability.
10.   F   Fads by definition are usually short-term behaviors.
11.   F   No particular food combinations as such have special therapeutic effects or facilitate weight management; body weight reflects energy balance.

Multiple Choice

1.   d   The food industry uses many food additives in processing foods to achieve multiple marketing goals. Some are good such as food safety and enrichment; others may be questionable.
2.   c   FDA has both monitoring and regulatory powers over food safety in all forms.

3.   d   The body requires specific nutrients found in a wide variety of foods, not specific foods as such.

4.   b   Factors such as agriculture, food availability, economics, marketing, distribution, and symbolic food meanings are cultural influences on food habits. Genetics exerts a physiologic influence on a person's reaction to various food factors and contributes to food tolerances.

5.   c   Kosher foods, according to religious laws, are those foods that avoid blood and meat-milk combinations.

6.   b   The Chinese method of stir-frying extends the use of small amounts of meat or fish and preserves the fresh flavor and texture of vegetables. The wok is designed to accomplish this task with very little fat.

7.   b   In the Mexican food pattern, corn is the most available grain; its lime-treated method of preparation over centuries has added valuable calcium to the diet.

8.   c   These five steps summarize a wise approach to follow in working with persons in any culture.

Chapter 10: Family Nutrition Counseling: Food Needs and Costs

Summary-Review Quiz

1.   11, 7, 14, 3, 11, 9, 11, 1, 11, 13
2.   5, 2, 8, 12, 4, 11, 6, 10, 11

3.   8, 4, 10, 1, 6, 5
4.   9, 2, 3, 7

5.   13, 6, 17, 3, 10
6.   1, 18, 8, 2, 15, 11, 5, 12
7.   7, 14, 4, 2, 16, 9

8.   11, 5, 1, 9
9.   9, 14, 3, 13, 7, 2, 10, 4, 12, 6, 8

10.   14, 5, 11, 1, 17, 10, 20, 2
11.   7, 12, 3, 19, 8, 16, 4, 18, 6, 13, 9, 15

Self-Test Questions

<u>True-False</u>

1. **T** Attitudes we form from all our life experiences are the basis of our behavior.
2. **F** Our brains can take in only a fraction of the multiple messages bombarding our senses constantly.
3. **T** This small percentage reflects how little we are trained to really listen in our highly competitive action-oriented American culture.
4. **T** Cooperative action in any situation is usually fostered by open discussion of reasonable goals and needs.
5. **F** Food value of meat relates to its nutrient value and leanness, not to its cost or texture, which are governed by marketing factors.
6. **F** The shell color has no relation to egg quality or food value.
7. **F** Removal of cream portion of milk affects only the fat value; protein remains in the non-fat portion.
8. **T** Various yellow and green vegetables and fruits supply the vitamin A precursor beta-carotene; citrus fruits and certain other fruits and vegetables supply vitamin C.
9. **F** Grades are not based on food values, but on other food characteristics of appearance.
10. **T** Whole grains contain many nutrients as well as energy and fiber; enriched grains have added B-vitamins and iron.

<u>Multiple Choice</u>

1. **a** This basic purpose is best achieved by actions that provide support for developing individual strengths, not ones that give false assurance and build dependent attitudes.
2. **c** Acceptance does not necessarily mean approval of a person's behavior but a valuing of individual integrity and a willingness to explore with a person the meaning of that behavior.
3. **d** All of these factors are part of human communication.
4. **b** Each of these responses may be used at various appropriate times in counseling interviews.
5. **c** These items are usually ones recorded in the patient's chart after a clinic visit.
6. **d** This type of question is more likely to obtain a valid useful answer for objectively exploring food habits. The other statements are judgmental and may well antagonize persons.
7. **d** This response is simply an objective summary reflection of a patient's statements. The other statements are judgmental and misleading.

Chapter 11: Nutrition During Pregnancy and Lactation

Summary-Review Quiz

1.   12, 5, 14, 3, 9
2.   1, 7, 13, 2, 11, 4, 8, 10, 6

3.   10, 2, 1, 14, 5, 7, 3, 13
4.   8, 6, 12, 9, 11, 4

5.   6, 12, 1, 6, 9, 14
6.   3, 11, 2, 13, 4, 8, 7, 8, 5, 10

7.   11, 4, 1, 9, 6, 8, 2, 12, 7
8.   3, 10, 5, 13

9.   13, 4, 9
10.   2, 14, 7, 1, 2, 11, 8, 5, 2, 7, 12, 3, 6, 10

11.   9, 5, 12, 3, 7, 6, 9
12.   1, 11, 2, 10, 4, 8

13.   7, 5, 1, 10, 4
14.   3, 9, 2, 6, 8

15.   9, 5, 12, 1, 11
16.   2, 6, 10, 4, 8, 7, 3

17.   12, 4, 1, 13, 6, 8, 2, 10, 9, 2, 10, 3, 11, 14, 10, 2, 5, 7

18.   8, 3, 10, 1, 9, 6, 5, 2, 7, 4

Self-Test Questions

<u>True-False</u>
1.   **T**   The mother's diet must supply the added nutritional demands of fetal development.
2.   **F**   This "parasite" theory is false; maternal diet must be nutritionally adequate for both fetal and maternal needs.
3.   **F**   This "instinct" theory is false; the mother eats according to learned foods habits, cultural attitudes, and knowledge of sound prenatal nutritional needs.

4. F Strict weight control during pregnancy is dangerous to both mother and child; sufficient weight gain is needed to support the pregnancy.

5. F Adequate sodium is needed for electrolyte balance given the mother's normally increased total body water during pregnancy.

6. T At both ends of the reproductive cycle, the mother is more at risk for developing pregnancy complications because of extremes of maturity of reproductive function.

7. F The successful outcome of any pregnancy is directly related to the mother's enhanced diet of good nutrition in supplying the necessary energy and building materials.

8. T The mother's increase in total body water, especially increased circulating blood volume, is necessary to handle the increased metabolic workload.

9. F This amount of gain is usually insufficient to support a normal pregnancy. Optimal weight gain is highly individual according to need; more problems occur with insufficient gain than with larger amount.

10. T Formation of bone tissue requires the major body mineral calcium.

11. T Daily iron intake is increased during pregnancy to help meet increased demand and avoid the "dilution" anemia related to increased blood volume and body water.

12. T Vitamin C needs for the integrity of tissue structure are enhanced during pregnancy.

13. T Vitamin D hormone is essential for absorbtion and use of calcium and phosphorus in bone-building.

14. F Pregnancy increases the need for folate; a deficiency causes megaloblastic anemia.

15. T Production of milk, a fluid tissue, requires adequate fluid in the mother's diet.

Multiple Choice

1. b All of these factors reflect the nutritional demands of pregnancy.

2. d Pregnancy is a prime example of biologic synergism reflected in the close interdependent functions of fetus, placenta, and the whole maternal organism.

3. a Blood volume increases 20% to 50% during pregnancy to support the increased metabolism.

4. d Optimal increases in all these tissues are normal in a healthy pregnancy.

5. b Only animal proteins are complete because they have all 9 essential amino acids.

6. c Increased maternal blood volume and fetal iron stores require added iron; fetal bone structures require more calcium and phosphorus along with vitamin D hormone. Menses cease during pregnancy.

7. b Liver is by far the highest dietary source of iron.

8. d Carrots supply the vitamin A precusor beta-carotene. Egg yolk and cream supply preformed vitamin A; citrus fruits supply vitamin C.

9. c   Multiple, relatively dry small snacks of carbohydrate foods are better tolerated during periods of nausea.

10. d   Increase in fluids and naturally laxative foods—those with high fiber content—and dried fruits such as prunes help prevent constipation. Use of laxatives can be dangerous during pregnancy.

11. c   All of these symptoms characterize pregnancy-induced hypertension (PIH), formerly called toxemia.

12. a   Pregnancy-induced hypertension (PIH) is closely related to malnutrition and poverty, both of which are associated with lack of prenatal care.

13. c   A lack of adequate circulating blood volume, or hypovolemia, results from abnormally low plasma protein, mainly albumin, needed to maintain the normal capillary fluid-shift mechanism for guarding vascular volume and ensuring tissue fluid circulation to nourish cells.

Chapter 12: Nutrition For Growth and Development

Summary-Review Quiz

1.   9, 6, 12, 3, 7, 1, 10, 2, 5, 8
2.   11, 4

3.   12, 4, 8, 14, 1, 7, 2, 10, 13, 3, 6, 9, 5, 11

4.   9, 3, 6, 1, 10, 2
5.   5, 5, 8, 7, 4

6.   10, 2, 6, 7, 1, 5, 9, 8, 3, 4, 7, 9

7.   11, 4, 14, 7, 8, 10, 1, 2, 12
8.   9, 3, 13, 6, 5

9.   5, 1, 7, 9, 12
10. 2, 8, 10, 3, 11, 6, 4

11. 4, 7, 1, 2, 6, 10, 3, 8
12. 5, 9

Self-Test Questions

<u>True-False</u>

1.   F   Infants and toddlers require adequate amounts of the essential fatty acid, linoleic acid, for normal growth; a main source of this essential nutrient in their diet is the cream portion of milk.

2. F Complete protein foods—milk, egg, cheese, meat—provide the essential amino acids. Adequate carbohydrate is needed for energy and protein-sparing.

3. T These three trace elements play roles in hemoglobin formation and tissue growth.

4. F Iron is needed for hemoglobin formation; calcium is needed for bone structure and maintaining serum calcium levels.

5. T Milk lacks iron; added solid foods such as enriched cereal, egg yolk, vegetables, and meats are needed after six months of age to supply needed iron.

6. F Vitamin C is water-soluble and any excess is excreted. Hypervitaminosis A and D may occur when the early supplement, usually given in concentrated drops, is given in spoon measures through ignorance or carelessness.

7. F Breast milk is uniquely adapted from early colostrum to mature milk to meet infant needs, including preterm, term, and older infants.

8. T The sucking of the infant stimulates these specific hormones to cause the "let down" reflex of milk flow.

9. F Newborn rooting and sucking reflexes are inborn to ensure food intake for survival.

10. T Required nutrients, energy, and fluids produce milk and supply infant needs.

11. T Different muscles and reflexes are required for eating solid foods from those needed for sucking milk.

12. F The growth rate after infancy slows and toddlers require less food in relation to body size. About a pint of milk in small ½ cup servings, or other equivalent dairy foods, will suffice.

13. T This natural monthly iron loss needs to be offset by use of iron-rich foods in the diet.

14. T The one function of iodine is to form thyroid hormone, the need for which increases during puberty to meet basal metabolic needs.

Multiple Choice

1. a Water-soluble vitamins and water-soluble amino acids (as all amino acids are) are not related to dietary fat. Dietary fat supplies fuel for energy, fat-soluble vitamins, and essential fatty acids.

2. d All of these protein-related needs are essential for the tissue protein synthesis of normal growth. A metabolic pool of amino acids supported by a sound diet ensures this supply.

3. a All of these functions require calcium.

4. c Iron-deficiency anemia is a relatively common childhood problem, as population surveys reveal.

5.   b   Pre-adolescent growth of girls exceeds that of boys; increased growth rate and sexual maturation occurs in all adolescents. All children gradually grow away from parental food habits to those of their social group.

Chapter 13: Nutrition For Adults: Early, Middle, and Later Years

Summary-Review Quiz

1.   6, 14, 10, 11
2.   8, 2, 9, 4
3.   3, 13, 7, 1, 5, 12, 11

4.   5, 7, 12, 2
5.   10, 1, 9, 4, 11, 3, 8, 6, 3

6.   11, 5, 7, 1, 9, 3, 12, 2, 8, 6, 10, 4

7.   5, 8, 12, 1, 10, 3, 9, 6, 2
8.   11, 4, 7

Self-Test Questions

True-False

1.   T   Physiologic and psychosocial needs differ in these two groups of older adults.
2.   F   In comparison with some other cultures, Americans generally devalue older persons as productive, contributing members of society.
3.   F   Much yet needs to be known about chronic diseases of aging, and generally medical and social care of the aged is poor.
4.   F   A gradual decrease in organ system capacities begins about age 30, but this course of aging is highly individual.
5.   T   This level of energy intake is average for adults, but individuals vary in need.
6.   T   Weight for height is basic index for energy balance.
7.   F   The absolute amount generally does not increase with age, but the relative amount (proportion of total kilocalories) may since the total caloric need may be less in comparison with more active younger years.
8.   F   Not necessarily, but some individuals may need them for specific helath reasons.
9.   T   Older persons are particularly vulnerable to fads because they wish to retard aging or because they have some health problem.

Multiple Choice

1. a   As a population, Americans are growing in number and increasing in age.
2. d   These needs largely summarize those of older adults.
3. d   Biologic aging is basically a process of gradual loss of cells and their related organ function.
4. a   With aging, an organ system's function after a stress load generally takes longer to return to normal because gradual cell loss causes reserve capacity to slowly diminish. The rate at which these changes occur, however, is highly individual.
5. a   Adult protein needs are related to biologic value of protein foods used, a sufficient caloric (energy) value of the diet to spare protein, and the person's health status, not to kind of fat used.
6. b   All, or any one, of these factors may limit food intake and contribute to nutritional problems in older persons.
7. d   All of these actions are wise ways of helping elderly persons with health problems while respecting and supporting their personal integrity.

Chapter 14: Nutrition and Physical Fitness

Summary-Review Quiz

1.   9, 3, 6, 9, 1, 10
2.   5, 2, 8, 7, 4, 9

3.   10, 6, 1, 8
4.   4, 12, 10, 9, 3, 7, 11, 5, 2

5.   9, 3, 9, 6
6.   4, 1, 10, 7, 9, 8, 5, 2

7.   14, 6, 18, 1, 9, 16, 2, 10, 5
8.   12, 7, 11, 8, 17, 3, 15, 4, 4, 17, 13, 4, 17

9.   12, 5, 14, 1, 10, 7, 7, 2, 8
10. 12, 13, 3, 9, 1, 13, 6, 11, 4

11. 11, 6, 2, 14, 1, 10, 4, 10, 12, 3, 8
12. 11, 7, 9, 13, 5

Self-Test Questions

<u>True-False</u>
1.   **F**   Cold water is the best replacement for water loss during normal sports and exercise; electrolytes are replaced by diet. However, heavy endurance exercise over longer periods of time may require an addition of glucose to the sports drink.
2.   **T**   Cold water is the best water replacement form because it is absorbed quickly.
3.   **F**   Drinking water before or during athletic events has not been shown to cause cramps; to the contrary, it helps prevent dehydration from water loss.
4.   **F**   Protein is not a fuel substrate for energy during exercise; carbohydrate and fat are.
5.   **F**   Vitamins and minerals are not energy compounds themselves; they act as coenzyme factors to regulate energy metabolism of fuel compounds.
6.   **T**   Carbohydrates provide glycogen stores.
7.   **T**   Evaporation of sweat from skin surfaces removes body heat, but in prolonged exercise more heat is generated so more water is lost and more water intake (not depending on the normal thirst mechanism) is essential to prevent dehydration and maintain body temperature.
8.   **F**   Exercise effects: improved circulation and oxygenation of blood improves heart disease, and increased number of insulin receptors improves diabetes.
9.   **T**   This level is needed for aerobic effect.
10.   **T**   Yes, but it must be brisk and maintained for a sufficient length of time.

<u>Multiple Choice</u>
1.   **b**   Swimming usually forces one into an aerobic level, whereas golf, tennis, and baseball are usually slower paced (when played by non-professionals).
2.   **d**   To have aerobic effect, exercise must sustain the necessary heart rate (70% of maximum) for the required length of time (20 to 30 minutes) and be practiced regularly to build up to this effect and maintain it.
3.   **d**   All of these factors are important. If you don't enjoy it, you won't continue it. It must be done regularly to be efffective and it must be done in moderation and not to harmful extremes.
4.   **b**   Increased insulin receptor sites from exercise in persons with non-insulin dependent diabetes mellitus (NIDDM) helps them to use better their endogenous insulin, as well as to control weight.
5.   **a**   Exercise helps regulate appetite by mobilyzing fatty acids for a fuel base and reducing stress. It also increases basal metabolic rate and lowers the "set-point" for fat deposit.

6.   c   Beneficial effects of exercise on bone are reduced bone weakness because of increased bone mineralization and decreased calcium withdrawal from increased muscle tension on bone. The overall result is increased bone density and strength.

7.   c   More sustained energy comes from complex carbohydrates (starches) and the resulting glycogen and glucose resources. Large heavy amounts of protein and fat drain energy for prolonged digestion and absorbtion and do not provide initial fuel substrate.

8.   a   Adequate protein, moderate fat, and liberal carbohydrate (especially complex forms) provide the best diet for supporting physical activity.

Chapter 15: Nutrition and Stress Management

Summary-Review Quiz

1.   9, 19, 3, 4, 12, 17, 1, 11, 6, 2, 16
2.   3, 15, 18
3.   13, 8, 5, 14, 10, 7

4.   8, 3, 10
5.   6, 9, 1, 7, 11, 5, 4, 2

6.   17, 5, 2, 13, 1, 15, 8, 11, 3
7.   18, 10, 4, 19, 12
8.   7, 16, 19, 6, 9, 14

9.   13, 9, 12, 9, 5
10.   1, 15, 7, 17, 3, 6, 11, 2
11.   16, 14, 8, 4, 10

12.   7, 9, 4
13.   1, 3, 8, 2, 6, 10, 5

14.   14, 10, 8
15.   6, 2, 13, 5
16.   1, 12, 9, 3, 4, 11, 7

Self-Test Questions

True-False

1.   F   Specific stressors cause varying responses in individuals, depending on different personal conditioning factors.

2.	F	The modern environment does not allow for former primitive responses and the repressed physiologic effects often cause illness.
3.	T	Normal physiologic stress always accompanies change.
4.	T	Prolonged stress must have adaptive relief to avoid exhaustion, illness, or eventual death.
5.	F	Personal perception of pain levels, tolerances, and feelings about health and disease are highly individual and cannot be precisely measured.
6.	T	Such adaptive homeostatic mechanisms help maintain life in balance with the environment.
7.	F	Psychosocial stress-coping mechanisms are learned mental/psychologic defense responses.
8.	F	Individual responses to stress vary widely according to personal situations and needs.
9.	T	Emotional tension, induced by a wide variety of life situations, is by far our most common modern human stressor.
10.	T	Any life stressor is always modified by its nature and duration, and the person's inner coping strengths.

Multiple Choice

1.	c	Instant transmission of initial stress alarms by this immediate 2-track system is vital for the quick physiologic defensive responses to sustain life.
2.	a	Hormones, hypothalamus releasing factor and catecholamines (epinephrine or norepinephrine) are the immediate chemical messenges; stored tissue fuel release results for defensive energy needs.
3.	d	All of these actions are normal physiologic responses to defend the body from stress effects.
4.	c	Return of neuroendocrine hormonal blood levels to normal are later effects of the initial resistance/adaptive response to stress.
5.	d	All of these stress factors describe body effects when stress-coping resources become exhausted.

Chapter 16: Nutritional Assessment and Therapy in Patient Care

Summary-Review Quiz

1. 4, 9, 14, 1, 11, 8, 2
2. 7, 3, 13, 6, 10, 5, 12

3. 16, 9, 12, 4, 20, 1, 18, 6, 11, 3, 19
4. 13, 7, 2, 15, 8, 5, 14, 10, 17

5. 7, 5, 1, 10, 8, 2
6. 4, 9, 6, 3

7. 4, 10, 14, 6
8. 1, 8, 12, 3, 2, 13, 5
9. 6, 11, 9, 7

10. 7, 11, 4, 12, 14, 1, 9, 8
11. 2, 13, 6, 3, 8, 5, 10

Self-Test Questions

<u>True-False</u>
1. **T** A person's plan of care must be based on full assessment of individual needs.
2. **T** Children especially need close attention to ensure adequate food and fluid intake.
3. **T** Hospitalization produces anxiety in most patients, and sometimes their defenses interfere with treatment, so they need much supportive care and exploration of real needs.
4. **T** Staying close by and having family present is helpful.
5. **F** It may even have contributed to the illness or posed problems in follow-up care.
6. **F** Patients are more often intimidated by the usual hospital setting and staff and often have little voice in their own care.
7. **T** A comprehensive history is one of the most valuable assessment tools in planning valid patient care.
8. **F** Social history is particularly helpful in understanding individual patient concerns and needs.
9. **F** Care must constantly be evaluated and revised as indicated to meet needs.
10. **T** The comprehensive base of all nutrient needs must be considered at all times to provide optimal nutritional support.
11. **F** Personal goals are a fundamental concern in planning nutritional care.
12. **T** If weight loss is to be achieved, the obese person's energy input must be less than total energy expenditure.
13. **F** Large food portions usually have the opposite effect on ill persons of reducing appetite.
14. **T** All persons respond to personal attention and festive tokens.
15. **F** Usually a person's family must be involved for an on-going care plan to be successful.

<u>Multiple Choice</u>
1. **d** All of these factors relate to individual needs.
2. **c** The hospitalization experience is influenced by these factors.

3.   b   The nutrition history involves all these factors to supply needed data for planning care.
4.   c   For valid therapy, all of these items must be considered.
5.   d   This is a relatively low-protein diet level, so no amounts of protein foods would have to be controlled.
6.   a   Full liquid diet includes milk and semi-liquid or soft milk-based foods.
7.   b   Actions should always involve the patient to the maximum capacity possible and provide any needed support to that end.

Chapter 17: Drug-Nutrient Interaction

Summary-Review Quiz

1.   16, 9, 1, 13, 20, 2, 6
2.   11, 18, 3, 10, 14, 14
3.   19, 5, 17, 12, 8, 15, 7, 4

4.   9, 3, 12, 1, 6, 11, 2, 8
5.   5, 9, 10, 7, 4

6.   12, 3, 14, 8, 1
7.   7, 10, 4, 13, 5, 11, 2, 9, 6

8.   10, 5, 12, 2
9.   1, 7, 4, 9
10.   11, 3, 4, 8, 6

Self-Test Questions

<u>True-False</u>
1.   F   The abuse of this drug and its side effects have caused it to be removed from recommended treatment of obesity.
2.   T   This undesirable side effect poses a nutrition-related problem in its use in treating rheumatoid arthritis.
3.   T   This nondigestible fiber compound decreases food mass transit time through the intestine and limits nutrient absorption time.
4.   F   Cimetidine is widely used to treat gastrointestinal disorders such as peptic ulcers; its action reducing excess gastric acid secretions aids nutrient absorption.
5.   T   Mucosal irritation, anorexia, and reduced food intake from alcohol abuse all contribute to nutrient malabsorption.

6.   F   Neomycin causes mucosal tissue changes to inhibit absorption of fat and fat-soluble vitamins A, D, E, and K.   Vitamin D is necessary for absorption of calcium.

7.   T   Continuous aspirin use can cause low-level blood loss from intestinal mucosa irritation.

8.   F   Aspirin absorption is hindered by the presence of food; a large glass of cold water facilitates absorption and prevents irritation to the empty stomach lining.

9.   T   Oral contraceptives induce a "pseudo-pregnancy effect" and cause a greater demand for this vitamin and other vitamins—folate, B-$_{12}$, riboflavin, and C.

10. T   Charcoal broiling, for example, increases drug metabolism in the liver through increased enzyme activity.

Multiple Choice

1.   d   Elderly persons with chronic illness take more drugs and run the risk of more errors in self-administering them.

2.   b   Non-digestible bulk adds volume, a sense of fullness, and lack of desire for food intake.

3.   a   By facilitating a more normal gastric acid flow through its antisecretory action, cimetidine facilitates enzyme action and nutrient absorption.

4.   c   Potassium-losing diuretics can lead to depletion of the mineral through induced gastrointestinal losses and increased renal excretion.   Potassium deficiency is marked by muscle weakness.

5.   d   Coumarin is an antimetabolite to vitamin K; hence, vitamin K can act as an antidote.

Chapter 18: Feeding Methods: Enteral and Parenteral Nutrition

Summary-Review Quiz

1.   16, 9, 8, 11, 15
2.   13, 6, 3, 14, 12, 2
3.   6, 10, 17, 16, 4, 7, 11, 1
4.   5, 13, 3, 12

5.   23, 16, 25, 8, 11, 21
6.   8, 24, 13, 1, 27, 7, 20, 19, 10
7.   10, 17, 9, 4, 22
8.   18, 15, 5, 26, 2, 6, 12, 8, 14, 3

9.   18, 12, 9, 16, 1, 20, 24
10. 7, 14, 21, 11, 3
11. 22, 6, 13, 2, 23, 15
12. 5, 19, 10, 4, 17, 8

13. 11, 17, 14, 21, 7
14. 1, 23, 2, 13, 6, 26
15. 19, 3, 9, 22, 4, 8, 5
16. 24, 10, 25, 12, 16, 18, 20, 15

Self-Test Questions

<u>True-False</u>

1.   **F**   Questions concerning enteral nutrition support (ENS) do not center on its effectiveness as a feeding method, for this has long since been proved. Rather, questions center on the most appropriate individual formula, the preferred method of formula delivery, and causes and extent of possible tube-related complications.

2.   **F**   Despite the recent publicity concerning hospital malnutrition, the lack of consistent adequate nutrition to meet metabolic demands is increasingly recognized as a serious concern. Surveys show that about 50% of surgical patients and 44% of medical patients suffer significant protein-energy malnutrition, with elderly patients most vulnerable.

3.   **F**   Proper use of general energy-nutrient oral supplements is the first choice because their use carries little or no risk of any complicating infections. Tube feeding is the second choice if sufficient oral intake of high caloric food and supplemental formula is not possible because the patient is too ill or the hypermetabolic demand is too great.

4.   **F**   Because blender-mixed formulas of regular foods carry a much higher risk of bacterial growth, cannot be fed easily through modern small-bore tubes, and present digestion and absorption problems, they are rarely, if ever, used now. Standard and special commercial formulas are regularly used to provide a sterile homogenized solution for the more comfortable small-bore tubes and ensure a calculated profile of intact or predigested nutrients.

5.   **T**   Fat delivers more than twice the amount of energy (kcalories) per gram than the other main energy component glucose, thus helping to meet the increased energy need and preserve protein for its essential tissue-building role.

6.   **T**   Venous catheters inserted surgically into specific veins for feeding basic nutrients in predigested elemental forms have provided a major advance in critical patient care.

7.   T   Because it indicates current nutritional status, PAB has become a major screening and monitoring test for use with TPN, whereas serum albumin measure (half-life of 21 days) gives long-term data concerning recent malnutrition.

8.   F   Both measures are major monitoring procedures, especially kcalories as a total energy measure to meet hypermetabolic requirements and preserve protein as the essential nitrogen source for combatting catabolism and rebuilding tissue.

9.   F   This used to be true with former products and equipment, but now with advanced technology, improved lipids may be combined with the glucose and amino acid base and called a 3-in-1 admixture. With additional molecules of electrolytes, vitamins, and adequate fluids, the whole feeding is called a total nutrient admixture (TNA).

10. F   Caution is needed in adding minerals to the TPN solution due to incompatibilities of certain elements and a tendency to form insoluble substances that separate out. Iron is not routinely added.

Multiple Choice

1.   b   The nutrition support team clinical dietitian, with advanced academic degree and clinical training, and certified in enteral and parenteral nutrition support by qualifying examination, is the team nutrition specialist, responsible with the team physician for each referred patient's nutrition assessment and management of nutritional therapy, in accordance with team protocol and team case conferencing.

2.   d   Each of these key team specialists has an essential responsibility for strict aseptic technique and infection control as indicated.

3.   d   For each of these reasons, home enteral tube-feeding is useful in continuing nutrition support.

4.   c   The most successful education programs for home ENS have followed the pattern described in the text. The teaching team of clinical dietitian and nurse usually conducts the patient and family education program prior to hospital discharge with follow-up home visits. The team pharmacist may assist in a session on formula preparation and drug administration via tube.

5.   b   Home TPN is successful only with carefully selected trained patients and their families. It is far more expensive than ENS and carries more risk of complications.

Chapter 19: Gastrointestinal Problems

Summary-Review Quiz

1. 8, 5, 1
2. 10, 3, 2, 9, 6, 4, 7

3. 11, 6, 14, 8, 4, 2, 9, 12, 10, 3, 7, 13, 1, 5

4. 12, 6, 15, 1, 9, 4, 16, 3, 8
5. 2, 13, 7, 11, 14, 10, 5

6. 8, 5, 1, 10, 3
7. 8, 6, 2, 4, 9, 7

8. 14, 3, 8, 1, 16, 10, 13, 6, 12
9. 9, 4, 1, 11, 5, 17, 5, 7, 2, 15, 18

10. 9, 4, 5, 1, 7, 2, 10, 4, 6, 5, 3, 8
11. 8, 5, 9, 1, 7, 3
12. 6, 2, 4

13. 9, 3, 6, 10, 8, 5
14. 1, 7, 2, 4

15. 7, 14, 13, 10, 4, 4, 1, 9, 2, 11, 8, 5, 12, 6, 3

Self-Test Questions

<u>True-False</u>
1. **T** The reduced incidence of dental caries is largely the result of fluoridation of public water supplies.
2. **T** This diet eliminates the need for chewing.
3. **F** Food trapped in a hiatal hernia is easily regurgitated when the person lies down.
4. **T** The resulting symptoms are clear, but the precise underlying cause of the abnormal secretory process or tissue sensitivity is not.
5. **F** Persons who develop ulcers do tend to be under stress, but this is not always the case.
6. **F** Pain occurs more when the stomach is empty; food buffers excess acid.
7. **T** Excluding gross individual irritants, regular foods provided in a supportive environment have proved to be far more effective than have highly restrictive bland diets of the past.

8.   F   A high-residue diet has eliminated symptoms even in hospitalized patients with active disease.

9.   F   Serious dehydration and potassium loss can occur in prolonged infant diarrhea.

10.   T   These foods are all sources of gluten, a part of which (gliadin fraction) is the agent causing celiac-sprue in sensitive persons.

11.   T   The genetic disease phenylketonuria (PKU) is caused by a lack of the cell enzyme phenylalanine hydroxylase, so these infants cannot metabolize the amino acid phenylalanine.

12.   F   Phenylalanine is an essential amino acid necessary for normal growth, so it cannot be eliminated from the diet but is limited according to individual tolerance levels.

13.   T   Lactose is not an essential nutrient (other dietary sugars can replace it), so a galactose-free diet can be used, eliminating all sources of lactose.

14.   T   Soybean-based formulas can replace regular milk formulas for children with milk allergies to supply all basic nutrients for growth.

Multiple Choice

1.   c   Control of acid erosion of mucosal tissue is a primary goal of both drug and nutritional therapy.

2.   d   This sequence of actions summarizes the essential nutritional therapy for infectious diarrhea.

3.   d   All sources of wheat are eliminated since it is the main source of gluten.

4.   b   Iron and folic acid are necessary for hemoglobin formation.

5.   d   These symptoms all reflect nutritional problems of ulcerative colitis caused by malabsorption and gastrointestinal losses.

6.   c   Sufficient kcalories and protein are necessary for tissue healing; supplements are needed to replace losses and prevent deficiencies. Milk is poorly tolerated.

7.   c   Lactase is the specific digestive enzyme for breaking down lactose.

8.   b   Hepatic encephalopathy in advanced liver disease is largely the result of ammonia intoxication; the failing liver cannot handle this nitrogen product of amino acid metabolism.

9.   c   All of these diet modifications may be used in the treatment of cirrhosis.

10.   a   High-fat foods trigger the cholecystokinin mechanism for bile release and cause pain at the wound site.

Chapter 20: Diseases of the Heart, Blood Vessels, and Lungs

Summary-Review Quiz

1. 10, 5, 1, 14, 3, 8, 7, 12, 2, 13, 11, 4, 9, 6

2. 5, 12, 9, 13, 1, 11, 3, 14, 2
3. 7, 1, 8, 1
4. 4, 10, 6

5. 10, 11, 5, 7, 2, 11, 1, 9, 4, 12, 8, 3, 6, 11

6. 4, 10, 16, 1, 11, 8, 2, 13
7. 15, 6, 7, 1, 14, 9, 3, 5, 12, 4

Self-Test Questions

True-False
1. **F** Heart disease incidence is greater in developed countries; it has been called "the disease of civilization."
2. **T** Such "workaholic" behavior strains heart disease-prone men to develop heart problems.
3. **F** Extremes of weight as well as degree of fatness pose health problems. Lean body weight without excess fat is desirable for health.
4. **T** The research focus on cholesterol and fat came from the early identification of the composition of these plaques.
5. **T** Statistical population surveys indicate greater incidence among blacks.
6. **T** The heart muscle tissue area cut off from its blood supply soon dies from lack of oxygen and nutrients.
7. **F** Cholesterol is an essential body substance, precursor for numerous life-sustaining materials such as vitamin D hormone and sex hormones.
8. **F** Because cholesterol is essential to life, the body constantly synthesizes an endogenous supply.
9. **T** This general term refers collectively to the various types of lipid disorders.
10. **T** This complex of fat and fat-related compounds packaged with a covering of water-soluble protein is necessary for transport in water-based blood.
11. **F** Saturation of fats makes them more dense, hence harder.
12. **T** This dietary fat imbalance is improved by reduction of animal fat in relation to unsaturated plant fat.
13. **T** Because of their relatively high content of cholesterol, eggs are limited on a low-cholesterol diet for hypercholesterolemia.

14. T   The injured heart muscle must be given an opportunity to heal by establishing collateral circulation around the affected tissue.

15. F   Coconut and palm oils are exceptions to the usual nature of food fat sources; although they are plant fats, they are saturated fats as are animal fats.

16. F   In congestive heart failure, the weakened heart muscle can no longer maintain the normal rate of action needed to handle the returning blood flow, so tissue fluid accumulates.

17. T   This mechanism, maintained by a balance of circulating fluid pressures, ensures constant nourishment of all body tissue cells.

18. T   With more sodium and water retained by aldosterone action, the problem of cardiac edema is increased.

19. F   The taste for salt in humans is a learned taste; sufficient sodium intake is present in the naturally-occurring mineral in foods.

20. T   When excess tissue sodium is reduced, a reduction in excess tissue water follows to maintain normal water-electrolyte balance.

21. F   Regular cheese has a relatively high sodium content, but low-sodium cheeses are available.

22. F   Essential hypertension has a genetic base; it is controlled, not cured, by diet and weight/stress control therapy aided by drugs as individually needed.

Multiple Choice

1. b   Chylomicrons carrying the fat load from meals are produced in the intestinal wall during absorption; the remaining endogenous lipoproteins are produced mainly in the liver.

2. c   Since chylomicrons carry the exogenous dietary fat from meals, they have the largest triglyceride and smallest protein composition of all the lipoproteins.

3. b   Liver and egg yolk are biologically designed to store cholesterol for their respective animal tissue metabolic needs.

4. c   All of these factors contribute to cardiac edema in circulatory problems and consequent fluid-electrolyte imbalance in congestive heart failure.

5. a   The natural seasonings do not contain salt or other sodium compounds such as monosodium glutamate (MSG).

6. a   Of all the food groups, fruits have the lowest natural sodium content.

Chapter 21: Diabetes Mellitus

Summary-Review Quiz

1.   16, 3, 18, 12, 7, 1, 9, 5, 14, 10, 18, 2, 17, 11
2.   8, 4, 20, 15, 19, 13, 19, 6

3.   11, 6, 14, 1, 9, 13, 4, 8, 3, 12, 2, 10, 7, 5

4.   9, 3, 6, 1, 6, 12, 7, 2, 1, 10, 6, 9, 11, 5, 8, 4

5.   14, 7, 18, 1, 16
6.   9, 11, 2, 5, 10, 17, 3, 12, 13, 8, 4, 15, 6, 9

7.   9, 3, 6, 1, 3, 10, 2, 8, 4, 7, 5
8.   10, 3, 7, 12, 1, 8, 6, 2, 11, 4, 9, 5

Self-Test Questions

True-False

1.   F   Persons with non-insulin-dependent diabetes mellitus (NIDDM) are usually obese adults.
2.   T   The female excretory anatomy and the constant heavy urinary glucose load provide an environment facilitating irritation and the growth of microorganisms.
3.   F   The energy balance nutrients most affected are carbohydrates and fats.
4.   F   Insulin is produced by specialized beta cells in the pancreas.
5.   T   These three hormones are interbalanced in regulating energy metabolism.
6.   T   This ketone is an intermediary product of fat breakdown and indicates an imbalance in carbohydrate metabolism.
7.   T   Self-monitoring of blood glucose has proved to be a great help to persons with diabetes, especially in NIDDM, in managing their necessary interbalance among food, insulin, and exercise to maintain normal blood sugar levels.
8.   T   Long-term diabetes predisposes blood vessels to atherosclerotic plaque development.
9.   F   Diabetes managed by a balanced diet that meets individual nutrition and weight needs, uses regular foods, and is adjusted as needed according to exercise and insulin activity.
10. F   No person, certainly not one with diabetes, should follow a low carbohydrate diet, which induces a deficiency of the body's main energy fuel.
11. F   NPH is a medium-acting insulin, covering about a 24-hour period.

Multiple Choice

1.   c   Conversion of glucose to fat is an irreversible action; fat is never converted to glucose.
2.   d   Normal insulin activity in controlled diabetes allows glucose to enter cells and participate in normal glucose metabolism to produce energy, or be converted to storage forms of glycogen and fat.
3.   c   Level of energy balance should be that which maintains ideal weight.

4. a   Meat and peanut butter are exchanges for cheese. Milk is in a separate group.
5. d   All these principles are incorporated in the exchange system of diet control.

Chapter 22: Renal Disease

Summary-Review Quiz

1. 6, 12, 7, 1, 9, 2
2. 11, 12, 8, 3, 10, 4, 7, 1, 5, 2

3. 3, 10, 6, 12
4. 1, 8, 14, 4, 14, 2, 11, 13, 9, 14, 14, 15, 5, 14, 7

5. 11, 7, 3, 1, 14, 5, 1, 8, 4, 2, 13, 10, 6, 12, 9

6. 12, 6, 8, 1, 2, 4, 16, 9, 15, 13, 10, 3, 5, 2
7. 11, 7

Self-Test Questions

True-False
1. T   Nephron function maintains normal levels of blood components.
2. F   Since they are so essential to life, an oversupply of hundreds of nephrons exist in the kidneys; only gradually are they reduced in normal aging.
3. F   Nephron action is basic to life because it maintains a normal blood supply and fluid-electrolyte/acid-base balance.
4. T   This tuft of capillaries cupped in a thin basement membrane at the head of the nephron tubules is specially designed to facilitate filtration of circulating blood.
5. T   These protein materials remain to maintain reabsorptive fluid balances for continuing circulation.
6. F   Most of the needed blood components are selectively reabsorbed in the first (proximal) section of the nephron tubule.
7. T   The main function of the narrow midsection is to establish the necessary sodium concentration to help concentrate the urine in the final distal tubule as it returns through this area for excretion.
8. T   Aldosterone causes sodium, hence water, reabsorption, thus contributing to urine concentration.
9. F   ADH is a water-conserving mechanism, hence it helps concentrate the urine.

10. **T** This necessary osmotic mechanism for concentrating urine is maintained by sodium pumps in the Loop of Henle.

11. **T** The resulting urine volume demonstrates the great concentrating power of the nephrons in guarding vital body water and its components.

12. **F** Since the acute disease is short-term and controlled by modern drug therapy, basic nutritional support is the primary goal.

13. **T** Replacement of the protein losses, with replacement protein supplement as needed, is a primary goal of nutritional therapy.

14. **T** In advanced renal disease, fewer and fewer functioning nephrons remain, bringing chronic renal failure.

15. **F** The loss of adequate nephron function brings numerous metabolic abnormalities and symptoms affecting not only nitrogenous substances such as urea, but also water, electrolyte, and acid-base balances.

16. **F** Low-protein products are necessary diet items.

17. **T** Normal muscle tension on bones is a necessary part of normal bone-serum calcium balance.

18. **F** Cystine is formed from its precursor, the essential amino acid methionine; hence dietary control of methionine is necessary.

19. **T** Increased loss of body water through sweat causes increased concentration of urine to conserve body water.

Multiple Choice

1. **b** Short-term acute disease requires normal protein and sodium for better nutritional support during healing, since modern drugs control the disease process.

2. **c** These abnormal blood and urine test results reflect the disease effect on the nephon's basement membrane and proximal tubule and the resulting loss of normal filtration-reabsorption capacity.

3. **d** All these metabolic problems result from loss of normal functions dependent on protein.

4. **a** Moderate protein with supplement as needed to replace loss, as well as sufficient kcalories, supply necessary nutritional support, and decreased sodium, in addition to protein, helps control edema.

5. **a** All of these symptoms reflect failing nephron function.

6. **d** These objectives are the basics of nutritional therapy for chronic renal failure.

7. **a** To meet these objectives, the needed diet modifications must reduce protein, supply sufficient non-protein kcalories for energy and protein-sparing, control the major water balance cations—sodium and potassium—and control water according to output.

8. **c** Diet treatment of calcium phosphate stones reduces the stone constituents and increases urine acidity to help control their reformation.

9.   a   Cystine (amino acid) stones are acid based and protein derived, so diet controls the cystine precursor amino acid—methionine—and decreases urine acidity.

10.   c   Uric acid is a product of purine metabolism; organ meats and concentrated meat juices are high sources of purines.

11.   a   Meat and milk products are main sources of phosphorus and calcium; fruits are not.

Chapter 23: Nutritional Care of Surgery Patients

Summary-Review Quiz

1.   4, 10
2.   1, 10, 7, 6, 2, 3, 9, 5, 8

3.   9, 5, 4, 8, 9, 1, 10, 8, 6, 8, 2, 3, 7

4.   13, 6, 10, 2, 1
5.   4, 14, 4, 12, 3
6.   9, 5, 7, 11, 8

7.   3, 6, 10, 9, 1, 7
8.   2, 8, 5, 4

9.   4, 11, 5, 9, 3, 12, 1, 5, 2, 8
10.   6, 10, 7

11.   16, 12, 9, 6, 1
12.   14, 3, 10, 5, 15, 13, 2, 8, 4, 7, 11

Self-Test Questions

<u>True-False</u>

1.   T   Food aspiration during anesthesia could be dangerous to maintaining a vital airway.
2.   T   Protein intake is necessary for wound healing and the prevention of extended catabolism.
3.   F   A period of negative nitrogen balance is common immediately after surgery because of protein losses and delayed protein intake.
4.   T   Water balance is essential for support of normal metabolic function and prevention of dehydration.
5.   F   This is the function of vitamin C, not vitamin D.
6.   F   Oral liquid formulas of high nutrient density can supply full nutritional support.

7.   **F**   Depending on amount of stomach removed, a gradual return to regular diet is indicated.

8.   **T**   This term describes the place and chemical action underlying the sequence of resulting symptoms.

9.   **F**   Fat loads continue to stimulate the cholecystokinin mechanism and cause pain.

10.   **F**   Feces formation differences at the respective ileum and distal colon ostomy sites cause different management needs and problems.

11.   **T**   Residue-free diet helps avoid need for fecal residue elimination so the wound area may heal.

12.   **T**   Vigorous individualized nutritional support is essential to the success of overall burn therapy during healing stages.

<u>Multiple Choice</u>

1.   **a**   Plasma protein, mainly albumin, balances with hydrostatic blood pressure to maintain the capillary fluid shift mechanism controlling the flow of circulating tissue fluids.

2.   **b**   Bone tissue is formed by the anchoring of the mineral matter to the protein matrix.

3.   **d**   Antibodies, blood cells, some hormones, and all enzymes are proteins; antigens are alien body invaders that these protein components of the immune system combat.

4.   **a**   An optimal supply of essential amino acids from complete proteins and/or elemental formulas is necessary for synthesis of tissue protein.

5.   **d**   All of these diet modifications are needed to control symptoms and ensure nutritional support.

6.   **d**   All these metabolic needs form the basis for optimal protein therapy supported by nonprotein kcalories in treating burns.

Chapter 24: Nutrition and AIDS

Summary-Review Quiz

1.   13, 6, 17, 9, 2, 15
2.   4, 18, 9, 11, 1
3.   5, 9, 3, 16, 10, 8, 9
4.   14, 7, 12

5.   7, 12, 4, 14, 2, 1, 10, 13
6.   3, 8, 5
7.   11, 9, 6

8.   5, 9, 1, 10
9.   7, 2, 6, 4, 8, 3

10. 5, 11, 17, 15, 8
11. 13, 19, 7, 16, 19, 3, 4
12. 1, 18, 9, 6, 10
13. 15, 8, 2, 14, 12

Self-Test Questions

<u>True-False</u>

1.   **T**   Although the patient may appear well in the early asymptomatic period, the disease process is increasing and its treatments or complications will begin to take their toll on the person's nutritional status.

2.   **T**   Initial weight loss, 10% or more of usual body weight, is an early part of the symptom-complex in the primary diagnosis of HIV infection. Though weight may seem stable during the extended "well" period, weight loss continues in spurts as the disease progresses, and serious body wasting from HIV infection then also becomes a cofactor in development of the full disease syndrome, as the malnutrition itself suppresses cellular immune function.

3.   **F**   This synthetic hormone similar to natural progesterone improves appetite and food intake, hence weight gain, in many AIDS patients, similar to the effects seen in cancer patients.

4.   **T**   Both of these factors lead to an "AIDS enteropathy" involving intestinal mucosal changes, blunting of villi and abnormal enzyme secretions that cause clinical malabsorption and decreased resistance to infection by opportunistic organisms.

5.   **F**   Hypermetabolism and altered energy metabolism, even increased resting energy expenditure, occurs in latter stages of AIDS, associated with increased body wasting and spread of opportunistic infections.

6.   **T**   Early positive nutritional intervention can help build nutritional reserves and provide sound nutrition guidelines for combatting the opportunistic illnesses and body wasting. Establishment of this personal professional relationship early in the disease provides a close source of ongoing nutritional counseling and support to help meet individual problems and personal needs as they occur.

7.   **T**   Given the nature and course of the disease process, and as yet no medical cure or vaccine to offer, the patient's comfort and treatment desires must play a major role in team care provided.

284

1.   c   Because the course of AIDS is currently a devastating and terminal illness, all care must center on the patient and maintain personal integrity, comfort, and support as much as possible at each stage.

2.   e   All of these client-centered actions are fundamental to any nutrition counseling, but they are particularly important for support of the AIDS patient.

3.   a   All viruses by nature are the ultimate parasites; they can only grow and develop in their hosts, require a specific antiviral drug, and are difficult to control.

4.   c   Although the three basic stages are experienced by all AIDS patients, individual disease course from initial infection to death may vary.

5.   a   This long relatively "well" period following infection has been deceptive and misleading to early investigators. Current research indicates that the virus has not gone away but is incubating and multiplying in special tissues, gathering strength to show its full effects in the final illness and death.

6.   d   All of these symptoms are common in the second stage of the disease course called AIDS-related complex (ARC).

7.   a   The whole course of the disease relates to the continuing retroviral destruction of special white cells (T cells) of the immune system by the HIV infection, until too few remain to protect against common diseases and death follows.

Chapter 25: Nutrition and Cancer

Summary-Review Quiz

1.   10, 6, 14, 1, 4, 12
2.   8, 13, 2, 7, 11, 9, 5, 3, 8

3.   9, 13, 1, 6
4.   14, 3, 11, 5, 2, 8, 7, 4, 12, 7, 10

5.   8, 4, 1, 10, 5, 9
6.   2, 6, 3, 7

7.   9, 3, 6, 1, 5, 10, 7, 2
8.   3, 8, 4

9.   8, 5, 1, 10
10.   2, 6, 9, 3, 7, 4

11.   12, 4, 8, 14, 1, 7, 10, 3, 13, 2
12.   11, 6, 9, 5

13.   9, 6, 3
14.   12, 1, 10, 4, 7, 11, 2, 8, 5

15.   12, 8, 1, 18, 5, 16, 3
16.   10, 7, 14, 9, 3, 17, 6, 15, 4, 6, 13, 11

Self-Test Questions

<u>True-False</u>
1.   **F**   Cancer cells arise from normal cells whose cell reproduction and growth has "gone wild" from lack of normal regulatory gene function.
2.   **F**   DNA is the master genetic control agent in the cell nucleus; RNA is its imprint messenger controlling specific protein synthesis in the cell cytoplasm.
3.   **T**   Chromosome threads are composed of successive lines of genes at specific sites.
4.   **T**   Substances that can alter the structure and hence control function of specific genes can cause cancer from the abnormal cell growth resulting.
5.   **F**   Connective tissue tumors are called sarcomas; carcinomas arise from epithelial tissue.
6.   **F**   In general, cancer is related to the tissue-aging process.
7.   **T**   For example, skin cancer has a genetic component but requires exposure to the sun's irradiation for development.
8.   **F**   Antigens are alien invaders (germs or cancer cells) that induce immune system responses to combat them.
9.   **F**   Problems in this neck-throat area are directly related to food texture and alternative feeding modes.
10.   **T**   Tyramines require monoamine oxydase (MAO) for their metabolism. When a drug action inhibits the action of this cell enzyme, food sources of tyramine must be controlled.

<u>Multiple Choice</u>
1.   **b**   Lymphocytes are special white blood cells that are major components of the immune system—T cells and B cells.
2.   **c**   Cyclophosphamide is an alkylating agent effective as an antineoplastic drug because it interferes with cell division by binding to DNA, RNA, and cell enzymes, preventing their normal cell reproduction actions.
3.   **d**   Unable to obtain energy from the basic fuel glucose, the body metabolizes its own tissues in a futile attempt to obtain alternative fuel sources.
4.   **a**   Special islet cells in the pancreas supply insulin.

5.	c	Primary losses of fluid and electrolytes from constant gastrointestinal circulation can lead to serious dehydration and metabolic imbalance.
6.	b	Epithelial cells of the mucosa have a short life and a rapid turnover.
7.	a	Increased dietary protein for tissue synthesis (anabolism) is necessary to counteract the ongoing tissue breakdown (catabolism).
8.	d	Soft, cold foods are generally more soothing to mouth problems and better tolerated than hot, spicy, or dry foods.

Chapter 26: Nutritional Support in Disabling Disease and Rehabilitation

Summary-Review Quiz

1.   1, 12, 6
2.   2, 7, 9
3.   8, 3, 11, 5, 10, 4

4.   9, 12, 5, 14, 7, 11, 2
5.   8, 1, 13, 3, 6, 10, 4

6.   10, 7, 5, 2
7.   7, 4, 9, 1, 6, 8, 3

8.   11, 6, 8, 4, 10
9.   1, 9, 5, 12, 11, 2, 7, 3

10.   10, 8, 11, 6, 5, 2, 9, 7, 3, 4, 1

11.   16, 11, 9, 18, 13, 6
12.   3, 19, 8, 3, 12, 1
13.   15, 15, 3, 17, 2, 7, 10, 2, 4, 14, 5

14.   13, 5, 10, 12
15.   5, 1, 3, 9, 4
16.   13, 7, 6, 11
17.   10, 8, 2

18.   12, 6, 8, 12, 4, 1
19.   10, 2, 13, 7, 5, 9, 14, 3, 11

20.   15, 4, 10, 1, 6, 2, 13, 9, 8, 3, 11, 16, 5, 14, 7, 12

Matching: Progressive Neurologic Disorders

1. c
2. a
3. e
4. g
5. b
6. d
7. f

Self-Test Questions

<u>True-False</u>

1. T   The multiple varied individual needs during post-injury/disease rehabilitation require closely coordinated team efforts.

2. F   The increasing number of disabled Americans, as the population increases and ages, strains government resources and financial cutbacks have occurred.

3. F   At forced work retirement at age 65, many previously healthy persons, especially men whose identity was tied to occupation, suffer disorientation and illness.

4. T   This is a realistic figure based on population projections, and warns of increasing personal social and financial strains.

5. T   This catabolic process after trauma follows distinct stages and requires nutritional intervention and support.

6. F   The increased metabolic work responses to injury demand increased energy resources.

7. F   Fat should supply about 30% of the diet's kcalories to provide the essential fatty acid, linoleic acid, and help yield sufficient energy.

8. T   Only special individual deficiencies or conditions may require specific doses of particular vitamins or minerals.

9. T   Independent living, to whatever degree is possible, is important to rebuilding self-esteem for disabled persons and requires personal and social support.

10. F   Rheumatoid arthritis, especially juvenile forms, may also affect internal organs such as heart and liver.

11. F   Osteoarthritis usually involves minor changes in hand joints; marked disability is uncommon.

<u>Multiple Choice</u>

1. e   The patient, along with the family, must always be the key focus of skilled and sensitive person-centered care, if maximum potential success of treatment is to be achieved.

2.   c   The number of disabled Americans is increasing and involves more elderly persons due to population increases and influence of chronic disease.

3.   d   These are the three basic goals of the rehabilitation process, more easily achieved with early continuous intervention.

4.   c   A high-protein, high-carbohydrate, and moderate fat diet best meets needs of the disabled person.

5.   d   Nutritional care for the person with rheumatoid arthritis varies with metabolic disease activity and requires careful and continuous consideration of all these factors.

6.   d   All of these conditions involve brain lesions affecting neuromuscular coordination.

DAILY FOOD INTAKE

Student_____

Date_____

Total Food Eaten (Check Carbohydrate Foods)	Fate of Carbohydrate Foods in the Body		
	Mouth	Stomach	Small Intestine

DAILY FOOD INTAKE

Student_____

Date_____

Total Food Eaten (Check Fat Foods)	Fate of Fat Foods in the Body		
	Mouth	Stomach	Small Intestine

DAILY FOOD INTAKE

Student_____

Date_____

Total Food Eaten (Check Protein Foods)	Fate of Protein Foods in the Body		
	Mouth	Stomach	Small Intestine

DAILY FOOD INTAKE

Student_____

Date_____

Total Food Eaten (Check Vitamin Foods)	Fate of Vitamins in the Body		
	Mouth	Stomach	Small Intestine

Tool A. Food Items Used According to Food Groups

Food Group	Items Used	How Prepared
Meat (including poultry and seafood)		
Other protein foods (eggs, milk, cheese)		
Fruits		
Vegetables		
Cereals, breads		
Seasonings		

Tool B. General Meal Pattern

Time	Place	Foods Used	Amount, Form, or Preparation
Morning			
Noon			
Evening			
Snacks			

Tool A. Food Items Used According to Food Groups

Food Group	Items Used	How Prepared
Meat (including poultry and seafood)		
Other protein foods (eggs, milk, cheese)		
Fruits		
Vegetables		
Cereals, breads		
Seasonings		

Tool B. General Meal Pattern			
Time	Place	Foods Used	Amount, Form, or Preparation
Morning			
Noon			
Evening			
Snacks			